learning disability nursing

2232

learning disability
nursing

Edited by

John Turnbull

Blackwell
Science

© 2004 by Blackwell Science Ltd
a Blackwell Publishing company

Editorial offices:
Blackwell Science Ltd, 9600 Garsington Road, Oxford OX4 2DQ, UK
    Tel: +44 (0)1865 776868
Blackwell Publishing Inc., 350 Main Street, Malden, MA 02148-5020, USA
    Tel: +1 781 388 8250
Blackwell Science Asia Pty Ltd, 550 Swanston Street, Carlton, Victoria 3053, Australia
    Tel: +61 (0)3 8359 1011

First published 2004

Library of Congress Cataloging-in-Publication Data

Learning disability nursing/edited by John Turnbull.
    p. cm
    Includes bibliographical references and index.
    ISBN 0-632-06463-3 (softcover: alk. paper)
    1. Learning disabilities–Nursing. I. Turnbull, John, RNMH

    RC394.L37L428 2003
    616.85'8890231–dc22
    2003061755

ISBN 0-632-06463-3

A catalogue record for this title is available from the British Library

Set in 10/12.5 pt Palatino
by DP Photosetting, Aylesbury, Bucks
Printed and bound in Great Britain using acid-free paper
by MPG Books Ltd, Bodmin, Cornwall

For further information on Blackwell Publishing, visit our website:
www.blackwellpublishing.com

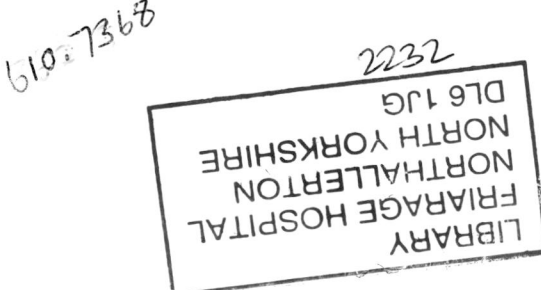

This book is dedicated to the memory of Stuart Crump,
a wise learning disability nurse, friend and colleague
who was taken from us too soon.

Contents

Preface

In recent years, learning disability nurses have embarked on two important journeys. The publication of *Valuing People* (Department of Health, 2001) the White Paper signalled the fact that we have entered a different and exciting era in the care and support of people with learning disabilities and their families. This is an era in which the emphasis will no longer be on where people live but how people live and, in particular, how they can be supported to exercise their rights and to lead full and satisfying lives. I firmly believe that learning disability nurses can play a key role in this future by using their distinctive knowledge and skill to work with individuals with learning disabilities, to provide support to families and other professionals and to influence the course of social change for the benefit of people with learning disabilities. If learning disability nurses are going to achieve this, they will need to develop their understanding of nursing practice and the sources of knowledge that nurses draw upon as well as make positive use of the factors that have combined to shape a learning disability nursing identity. A book like this might not be able to fulfil all of these needs but it was written to help learning disability nurses make a start on this journey. It was also written to help others understand learning disability nursing better so that they can provide support for their colleagues.

At the same time that services in which nurses work are undergoing change, there has never been a greater demand on professionals to account for their practice. Part of this means describing and explaining their practice to others in order to build trust and confidence. Part of this also means being able to demonstrate where success has been achieved. In the past learning disability nurses have had problems in describing and providing evidence of their contribution to people's lives. Therefore, this book was written to provide some signposts for nurses in their other journey into a future in which there will be clearer role expectations of learning disability nurses.

Given this, the contributors to this book and I hope that readers will use it to approach the future with greater confidence in their practice but ultimately in the expectation of healthier and more valued lifestyles for people with learning disabilities.

John Turnbull

Department of Health (2001) *Valuing People: A New Strategy for Learning Disability for the 21st Century*. Department of Health, London.

Contributors

John Aldridge Cert Ed, MA, RN (LD), RMN is a Senior Lecturer in Learning Disability Nursing at the University College, Northampton.

Peter Dawson RNMH is an independent self-advocacy worker.

Colin Doyle BSc, MSc, RNMH, Cert MHS is a Senior Clinical Nurse Specialist at St. Andrew's Hospital, Northampton.

Adrian Jones BA (Hons), RGN, RNMH is a Community Nurse for Children and Adolescents with Learning Disabilities, Sheffield Children's Trust.

Gwen Moulster MA, Cert Ed, RN (LD) is the Lead Nurse, Learning Disabilities Directorate, West Hampshire NHS Trust.

Sharon Pickering BA, BA (Education), Dip Health and Social Services Management, Dip. Nurs (London), MSc, RGN is the Head of Contracting and Training at the Trent Workforce Confederation.

Stephen Rawlinson BSc (Hons), RNMH, RMN, Dip Counselling is a Community Learning Disability Nurse at the Devon Partnership NHS Trust.

Tim Riding Dip HE, BSc (Hons), PhD, RNMH is the Network Lead for Secure Services at Lancashire Care NHS Trust.

Jackie Roberts Cert Ed, Dip Nurs, RNMH, NNEB, Cert Further Adult Education is a Senior Community Nurse at the Oxfordshire Learning Disability NHS Trust.

Jeanette Thompson BSc (Hons), Dip Nurs (London), PGDip (Management), Dip Health and Social Services Management, Cert Ed, MA, RNMH is a Lecturer in Learning Disability Nursing at the University of York.

John Turnbull BA, MSc, RNMH is the Director of Nursing at Oxfordshire Learning Disability NHS Trust and a Lecturer in Health and Social Care at the University of Reading.

Jill Turner BA (Hons), Dip HE, RN (LD) is a Lecturer Practitioner in Learning Disability Nursing at Oxford Brookes University and a Clinical Nurse Specialist at Oxfordshire Learning Disabilities NHS Trust.

Rebecca Welsh RN (LD), Dip Epilepsy Care is a Community Learning Disability Nurse at West Hampshire NHS Trust

Julie Wilkins RNMH, RMN is a Community Learning Disability Nurse at the Devon Partnership NHS Trust.

Chapter 1

Discovering learning disability nursing

John Turnbull

Introduction and aims of the book

This book is about learning disability nursing practice, how learning disability nurses experience it, and how it fits into the lives of people with learning disabilities and their families. Learning disability nurses have had to become familiar with thinking about and reflecting on their practice in the face of increased scrutiny of their role and the changes they have undergone (Turnbull, 1997). In spite of this situation, this book joins less than a handful of others that have been dedicated to exploring the role of the learning disability nurse. After nearly one hundred years of professional practice some might feel it curious, and possibly scandalous, that there is such a dearth of publications about this branch of nursing. As this introductory chapter will show, this situation can be explained by a number of inter-related factors such as how others have viewed their profession, how nurses perceive themselves and a lack of systematic enquiry into their practice.

Most professional groups working in the field of health and social care would claim that the general public, policy makers, managers and, sometimes, the people they serve do not fully understand what they do. However, it would not be an exaggeration to suggest that learning disability nursing is the most poorly understood profession amongst them. Therefore, one of the aims of this book is to promote understanding of the role of learning disability nurses. Added to this is the fact that, although countless learning disability nurses apply their knowledge skilfully and confidently in everyday practice, it can be difficult for them to gain a perspective on the breadth and depth of practice within the profession. This is important to help nurses articulate their role to others, as well as providing a platform for building knowledge about their practice and making sure that it remains relevant. Therefore, a second key aim of this book is to develop learning disability nurses' understanding of the aims of their practice, the knowledge they draw upon to inform their practice and how this combines to meet the needs and priorities of people with learning disabilities and the demands of the policy context in which they practice. Finally, although learning disability nurses are unique, they share a history that reveals common themes, and are subjected to the same assumptions about their role by others. For this reason a third aim of the book is to explore the identity of learning disability nurses and its impact on their practice.

The scope and structure of this book

When planning this book it became clear that, in order to achieve these aims successfully, there would need to be a focus on the day-to-day practice of learning disability nurses. Having realised this, the next key issue was to discover the best way of obtaining information about nursing practice. One option would have been to simply review the available literature. There are a small but growing number of nurses who have been prepared to write about their practice and, thankfully, an increasing number of journals in this specialist area to publish their work. There have also been a modest number of research projects into learning disability nursing. These would have provided a good source of information on which to reflect. However, it was decided not to use these sources as the *sole* foundation of the book. One of the reasons for this was that many of the published accounts of practice lack detail and insight into what it feels like to be a learning disability nurse, which is a key aspect of this book. Another reason was that the research projects have been inevitably carried out with certain aims and objectives and, therefore, could not cover the scope of this book. Therefore, it was decided to ask nine practising nurses to each write a chapter about their experiences in order to provide the reader with a greater insight into the aims and practice of learning disability nursing, as well as to provide information for the other contributors to draw upon in their more theoretical and reflective chapters.

When deciding whom to ask to contribute a practice chapter to this book, it quickly became evident that it would be undesirable, if not impossible, to try to include a representative sample of learning disability nursing practice. Not only is the breadth of practice too great but also every individual with learning disability and every context in which practice takes place is unique. Instead, the decision was informed by the editor's personal knowledge of the individuals and their high level of self-awareness that, in turn, enhances their ability to reflect upon and record their experiences. The nurses who were invited to contribute were asked to base their chapter on an individual or small group of individuals with whom they have worked and to write about an episode or an aspect of working with that individual that would, in their view, highlight an important facet of working as a learning disability nurse. The contributors were told that this could include episodes where their practice had not gone well because the aim of the book is to present a naturalistic picture of learning disability nursing rather than make judgements about what might be termed specialist, advanced or even best practice. Although such terms may be in common usage within nursing, there is little agreement about their meaning (Woods, 1997; Scott, 1998). Furthermore, a key aim of the practice chapters is to provide readers with an opportunity to reflect on the descriptions of practice. This would be made difficult if a judgement had already been made about their value through the attribution of a label. Because of this, care has also been taken over the titles of the practice chapters. The chapters have inevitably focused on specific topics when working with people with learning disabilities. For example, in Chapter 2, Tim Riding describes working with someone who has offended. In Chapter 4, Colin Doyle describes working with someone who displays challenging behaviour and, in Chapter 12, Rebecca Welsh writes about working with someone who has epilepsy. In spite of this, it is important to note that all of the practice chapters do not set out to present a blueprint of how to work with such individuals. The fact that some people have epilepsy, autism or display challenging behaviour is incidental to the central aim of describing the experience of practising as a learning disability nurse.

Naturally, a major concern was to preserve the identities of the individuals with whom these nurses worked. Therefore, the contributors have gone to great lengths to maintain anonymity by changing either the name, gender or age of the person as well as those who were also supporting or related to them. They have also modified the setting for practice and, in some cases, the point in time when their practice took place. Some contributors chose to present a composite picture of two individuals. Despite the fact that the contributors disguised the identity of the people they worked with, their accounts retain their value because they are taken from the actual experience of a learning disability nurse.

Because one of the aims of the book relates to how nurses experience learning disability nursing, the contributors to the practice chapters were asked to preface their description with a brief account of how they came to be a learning disability nurse and their motivation to work with people with learning disabilities. These revealed many common themes that will be taken up later in this chapter. Before moving on to describe the theory chapters, tribute must be paid to the authors of the practice chapters. Committing one's thoughts to paper is always a courageous act because others are then in a position to judge them. In this case, the contributors deserve further admiration because they have been prepared to expose their practice, as well as their thoughts, to scrutiny.

Deciding on the structure of this book was not easy. There was a need to break up the sequence of practice chapters by including chapters that could reflect on some of the key issues relating to learning disability nursing. The contributors to these chapters were asked to reflect on the relevant literature in the field as well as the content of the practice chapters in order to:

- Describe what it means to be a learning disability nurse.
- Describe what a learning disability nurse aims to achieve and what they do to help achieve these aims.

- Describe the relevance of learning disability nursing.
- Describe a framework for how to practice as a learning disability nurse.

These reflective chapters do not have to be read sequentially. In fact, all of the chapters in this book are designed to stand alone and can be read in any order. Even in cases where the theory chapters refer to events in the practice chapters this has been done in such a way that it is not necessary to have read the practice chapters first.

Aims of this chapter

As far as this chapter is concerned, it aims to explore the context and assumptions within which learning disability nurses practice, and asks whether they combine to create a learning disability nursing identity and, if so, what lies at the heart of this identity.

All professionals in the field of health and social care over the past two decades have faced common challenges to their professional aspirations and the way in which they practice (Southon and Braithwaite, 1998). This has included the need to account more thoroughly for their practice, the need to explicitly support their practice by the best available evidence and to ensure their practice represents good value for money. These issues have applied equally to learning disability nursing. Learning disability nurses will also share values such as compassion and altruism with their professional colleagues. However, there have a been a number of events, experiences and characteristics that combine in a distinctive way to shape the way that learning disability nurses feel about themselves.

Close relationships

Although many health and social care and educational professionals work with people with learning disabilities, learning disability nurses are the sole professional group that is educated specifically to work with them. This fact should not be underestimated because it forms the basis of how learning disability nurses think and feel about people with learning disabilities and how that explains their motivation and actions. Many learning disability nurses will say that they came into the nursing profession out of a motivation to work with people with learning disabilities rather than to become nurses. The nurses who wrote the practice chapters in this book explain the unique circumstances that brought them into the profession but the common theme is this desire to work with people with learning disabilities rather than a desire to be health care professional. Adrian Jones, in Chapter 11, says that he became a learning disability nurse to right the injustice to which he felt people with learning disabilities were subjected. Others, like Tim Riding in the following chapter, saw working with people with learning disabilities as stimulating, challenging and worthwhile. Jill Turner, in Chapter 3, touches on a common feeling amongst learning disability nurses that their work brings opportunities to get close to people and to work with them as individuals, without the barriers of uniforms and diagnostic tools.

Rebecca Welsh, in Chapter 12, describes another significant aspect of working with people with learning disabilities – that it can be life-changing for the nurse as well as the individual with learning disabilities. In Rebecca's case, her assumptions about people with learning disabilities changed profoundly as she came to see them as equals with a common humanity. However, it is also common for nurses to have their views changed about a whole range of issues and aspects of life through their practice experience. Richardson (1997) has described poignantly the reciprocal nature of nurses' relationships with people with learning disabilities when he celebrated the brief life of a person whom nurses had supported. Richardson makes the key point that nurses should *expect* to be changed by the experience of caring and supporting people with learning disabilities.

These examples describe the experience of *reciprocity*, which is defined as the process of learning from each other. *Mutuality* is a complementary process that can be understood as undergoing a common experience. This can take many forms. There is a theme within learning disability nursing that nurses are making a journey with people with learning disabilities. For some nurses, this is represented by the journey of people with learning disabilities, from being controlled and devalued, to becoming a citizen and accessing their rights. In Chapter 6, Peter Dawson's account of knowing Judith provides a microcosm of this journey and its struggles. There are parallels between his feelings of powerlessness as a nurse in the face of the hospital and Judith's powerlessness as a hospital resident. When Peter acquires a new post outside the hospital, he is in a better position to help her. Stephen Rawlinson, in Chapter 8, describes a process in which he was learning how to be a supportive facilitator for the tenants' group at the same time as his tenants were learning how to be a group.

Finally, Duncan Mitchell's research (1996, 1998, 2000) into the history of the learning disability nursing profession illustrates further examples of mutuality. Mitchell claims that learning disability nurses have suffered a loss of esteem because they have undergone a process of stigmatisation which parallels that endured by people with learning disabilities (Mitchell, 2000). There is no doubt that nurses have been marginalised, and even exploited, and these issues will be discussed at greater length later in this chapter. However, part of the reason for the stigmatisation endured by nurses is the simple fact that there is a general misunderstanding of learning disability itself, both by the public and the media (Philpot, 1995). In addition, professionals in health and social care themselves frequently display low levels of knowledge about learning disability (McKenzie *et al.*, 1999). If people do not have a concept of learning disability then they will be unable to imagine the type of care and support that people might need. The philosophical changes in the field of learning disability in recent years also play a role as far as nurses are concerned, in that they may be reluctant to tell the public that they are a nurse because they do not want to reinforce the impression that people with learning disabilities need medical care. The impact of this on learning disability nurses should not be underestimated. Although there are gender variations, a person's job, title and role plays a significant part in helping to develop that person's identity, and the public and profession's negative reactions to learning disability could be a source of frustration and a challenge to be met on a daily basis. Unfortunately, research has not explored this phenomenon or how nurses cope when it happens.

The pioneering spirit

The person-centred approach and strong commitment to people with learning disabilities that comes across in the practice chapters has perhaps provided the motivation for learning disability nurses to make some unique changes in their education and practice, showing their versatility and pioneering spirit. On a strategic level, for example, no other profession has undergone such a radical transformation in the setting in which their practice occurs. Learning disability nursing has moved from the hospital into the community. At an individual level, the impact of this transition is described eloquently by Stephen Rawlinson (Chapter 8) who entered into practice at a time when learning disability nursing in his area had only recently been moved into the community. Given the misgivings of some of his hospital colleagues, this must have required a good deal of courage.

The transformation of learning disability nursing has also been paralleled in terms of the aims of the profession. There have been occasions when the profession has had to revisit its value base and to develop a new vision for both the profession and a new system of education. One such occasion in 1982 is discussed in Chapter 5. At the present time, learning disability nurses are again revisiting their practice in the light of the new White Paper, *Valuing People* (Department of Health, 2001). In the next section, it will be seen that some learning disability nurses have had to give up their identity as nurses to practice in social care settings. It is questionable how many professions have members who would be prepared to do this but perhaps indicative of the loyalty that learning disability nurses feel towards people with learning disabilities.

The great divide

An issue that has created significant and unique problems for learning disability nurses is the distinction between health and social care. The NHS and

Community Care Act (Department of Health, 1990) introduced the need for a sharper distinction between responsibilities for health and social care needs within Health Authorities and Local Authority Social Services Departments. In the early years of implementing the Act, health care organisations seemed more concerned with demonstrating to authorities that they *weren't* providing social care, and vice versa, than they were about providing better quality care in line with their responsibilities. The newly formed NHS Trusts and the growing number of independent sector providers were encouraged to focus on their 'core business' in order to clarify and demonstrate accountability. This resulted in commissioning bodies, inspectorates and service managers spending much of their time policing the boundaries between health and social care rather than focusing on innovative and creative solutions to people's needs and wishes. The health and social care issue provoked considerable debate within the field of learning disability, and in other areas as well, where the focus for discussion was how professional practices could be linked with either 'health' or 'social' gain. Amongst learning disability nurses, there was a reluctance to talk openly and honestly about their skills because they found themselves in a dilemma – it was quite easy for them to demonstrate their contribution to both health and social care. However, given the atmosphere of the time, this would have given both health and social care organisations a good reason *not* to employ learning disability nurses. Although other professional groups faced difficulties over the health and social care issue, it was probably only learning disability nurses who had to suffer the indignity of having to play down the breadth of their skills and almost 'practice in disguise'.

In common with many other observers at the time, Cullen (Four Chief Nursing Officers, 1991) pointed out that the distinction between health and social care is largely an artificial one and that, in reality, people with learning disabilities, and the general public for that matter, have a mixture of needs. In more recent years, although Health and Local Authorities have still had to account for their respective spending on health and social care, there has been a greater recognition of the need for partnership between the two in order to help one another meet those needs.

Where this situation has had its greatest impact is on the employment status of learning disability nurses. For example, it is illegal for organisations to employ nurses to carry out social care functions. During the 1980s and 1990s the main alternative to hospital or health care provision became the residential care home. Nurses who had previously supported individuals in hospitals and wanted to continue to support them found themselves having to give up their status as nurses to work in these homes. The irony was that their aims, as nurses working with people with learning disabilities, had not changed and they were probably undertaking activities that could quite easily be construed as nursing (Turnbull and Timblick, 1998). It is understandable that learning disability nurses have felt great resentment about having to practice in what seems like a form of professional exile. As long ago as 1979, the Jay Report (Jay, 1979) recognised the contribution of learning disability nurses to day and residential services. More recently, Raynes *et al.* (1994) have shown how nursing skills are highly valued in social care settings. Although there is no suggestion that employers were unscrupulous, evidence such as this simply added to feelings of exploitation within the profession.

In response to the dilemmas facing nurses and their feelings of exploitation, Cullen (Four Chief Nursing Officers, 1991) recommended that nurses should promote their health care role. As Moulster and Turnbull point out in Chapter 5, nurses have incorporated more health care aims into their practice in recent years and their ability to accommodate them into practice in such a short space of time should be admired. On the other hand, as Moulster and Turnbull also point out, it is questionable whether learning disability nurses can be characterised as purely health care professionals, and the question remains about how open nurses are prepared to be about their practice. From a professional and educational point of view, this is an unhealthy position in which to be. At a strategic level, the development of joint training programmes, leading to a dual qualification in learning disability and social work, would give nurses the potential for greater flexibility in working in both health and social care settings (Brown, 1994a). For some nurses, this may have been a reality. For others, it did not change the fundamental problem that nurses could not openly utilise their nursing skills if they were employed in social care settings. Furthermore, although the dual qualification may have benefited individual nurses, it created potential problems for the profession as a whole because it gave nurses the opportunity of leaving the profession to work with other client groups.

An ambiguous relationship

Mitchell (1998) has already drawn attention to what he calls learning disability nurses' 'semi-detached' relationship with the more dominant adult branch of nursing. Amongst other examples, he describes how the nursing authorities were reluctant to admit learning disability nurses to the nursing register in the early part of the last century because their work was not perceived to be 'real' nursing. Nurses were eventually admitted to the register but events since then have reinforced learning disability nurses' beliefs that they are tolerated by the nursing community and would be sacrificed if it were in the interests of general nursing. For example, in 1972, the Briggs report (Department of Health and Social Security, 1972) recommended the abolition of the learning disability branch of nursing. In 1979, the Jay Report (Jay, 1979) agreed by recommending the phasing out of learning disability nursing and the creation of a new professional group to work with people with learning disabilities in residential facilities. None of these recommendations were put into practice but, at a consensus conference on the future of the profession in 1993, five options for the future education of learning disability nurses were proposed, only one of which entailed keeping the branch. The panel decision recommended keeping learning disability nursing in the family of nursing but as a post-registration specialty. However, after many in the profession and beyond expressed dissatisfaction with this recommendation (Brown, 1994b) the Department of Health abandoned the plan.

The fact that the Department of Health chose to retain learning disability nursing following these reports calling for its abolition has so far been interpreted in three ways. Ryan and Thomas (1980) believed that the failure of the Department to take up the recommendations of the Jay Report is that it lacked the political will to take on the trade unions and professional organisations that opposed the recommendations. Another explanation is that, far from wanting to marginalise learning disability nursing, the Department of Health, and successive Chief Nursing Officers in particular, have shown great leadership in saving the profession from the clutches of a managerial agenda that believes that health care would be a more ordered community with fewer professional groups (Birchenall, 1996). A third explanation is that prominent leaders and policy makers within nursing have used learning disability nursing to protect more valued members of the family of nursing. In other words, if powerful managers could save money by getting rid of a small branch like learning disability nursing who nobody seemed to be concerned about, then it would be easier to take on other specialties with greater prestige where there were more savings to be made, such as health visiting and school nursing.

The difficult relationship between learning disability nursing and general nursing also manifests itself over the issue of the generic nurse. Many people believed that the introduction of the Project 2000 system of nurse education, with its common foundation programme, was the beginning of a move to introduce a generic nurse. It could also be argued that the Jay Report and the consensus conference were also attempts to introduce such a nurse. Mitchell (2003) points out how difficult it is for nurses to practice whilst such a threat looms. Like a comet, the debate about the generic nurse will undoubtedly return and learning disability nurses will wonder how long it will be before they are obliterated.

It is important to recognise that the uneasy relationship between learning disability nursing and general nursing does not just exist at senior levels within the profession. For example, Turnbull (2002) pointed to the perennial problem of nurse lecturers from the adult branch of nursing telling learning disability nursing students to give up their branch programme because it had no future.

Finally, if the marginalisation of learning disability nursing has been perpetuated because it is thought that it does not conform to some sort of norm about nursing practice, then this hides a great irony. Far from being an eccentric member of the family of nursing, learning disability nursing is symbolic of the type of nursing to which many nurses would aspire. For example, learning disability nurses are engaged in social change, health promotion and public education. Furthermore, learning disability nurses no longer practice in the context of a subservient relationship to medical staff and they have learned how to take their knowledge and skills to wherever their clients live. Therefore, genericism may be a threat to the general nursing community and not just to learning disability nurses.

Given this history, it may be understandable that learning disability nurses feel resentment towards the adult nursing branch. However, learning disability nurses may not have been entirely innocent or fair in their dealings with their adult nursing colleagues. Earlier in this chapter it was pointed out that one of the strengths of learning disability nurses is the fact that their practice focuses on one particular group in society. Whereas this has a number of benefits, a disadvantage is that this could encourage an insular way of looking at nursing practice and a reluctance to look outside the field. For example, learning disability nurses can be reluctant to engage with and apply theoretical frameworks that have been developed within the sphere of general nursing. This is in spite of the fact that nursing models and theory can be adapted relatively easily to learning disability practice (Navrady, 1998; Spencer, 2002).

Problem or solution

The marginalisation of learning disability nurses has not only been caused by general nursing colleagues and nursing policy makers. Learning disability nursing has also been the subject of stereotyping from colleagues within the field of learning disability itself. For example, there are some who still believe that learning disability nurses work within a discredited medical model of care. This is almost certainly an assumption that developed from when nurses worked in the long stay hospitals, and it is surprising and frustrating to learning disability nurses that they have been unable to shake off this image. Jeanette Thompson and Sharon Pickering show in Chapter 9 that learning disability nurses do not deserve this reputation and that their practice remains relevant to the needs of people with learning disabilities, as well as to a number of practice imperatives.

There is another group of people within the field of learning disability who have raised questions about learning disability nursing practice and whom nurses have had to confront. These are individuals who see learning disability nursing as part of the problem faced by people with learning disability rather than part of a solution to help them lead more valued lifestyles. This is based on the belief that the very provision of specialist support such as learning disability nurses adds to the stigma and oppression endured by people with learning disabilities (Dowson, 1997).

Conclusion

The discussion in this chapter has suggested that learning disability nursing has an identity, which is comprised both of assumptions that learning disability nurses have generated about themselves and from how others perceive them. This identity cannot be reduced to a single sentence definition but any attempt to describe it would include reference to a struggle for recognition and acceptance within the field of learning disability, as well as feelings of marginalisation and exploitation. This has often led to learning disability nurses feeling unconfident and reluctant to speak out. At the same time, the learning disability nursing identity can also be defined by the creativity and flexibility that nurses show both at a strategic and individual level. It is highly probable that there is a causal relationship between the negative and positive features of the learning disability nursing identity. This could be an interesting avenue for future research.

References

Birchenall, P. (1996) Learning disability nursing: developing new horizons. *Nurse Education Today*, **16**, 83–4.

Brown, J. (1994a) *The Hybrid Worker*. University of York, Department of Social Policy and Social Work, York.

Brown, J. (1994b) *Analysis of Responses to the Consensus Conference Panel's Decision on the Future Education of Learning Disability Nurses*. University of York, Department of Social Policy and Social Work, York.

Department of Health (1990) *NHS and Community Care Act*. Department of Health, London.

Department of Health (2001) *Valuing People: A New Strategy for Learning Disability for the 21st Century*. Department of Health, London.

Department of Health and Social Security (1972) *Report of the Committee on Nursing*. HMSO, London.

Dowson, S. (1997) Empowerment within services: a comfortable delusion. In Ramcharan, P., Roberts, G., Grant, G. and Borland, J. (eds) *Empowerment in Everyday Life: Learning Disability*. Jessica Kingsley, London.

Four Chief Nursing Officers (1991) *Mental Handicap Nursing in the Context of 'Caring for People'*. Department of Health, London.

Jay, P. (1979) *The Report of the Committee of Enquiry into Mental Handicap Nursing and Care*. HMSO. London.

McKenzie, K., Murray, G., Matheson, E., Higson, J. & Sinclair, B. (1999) What is learning disability: do people need to be reminded? *Learning Disability Practice*, **2**(1), 8–11.

Mitchell, D. (1996) Learning disability nursing in the post war period. *International History of Nursing Journal*, **1**(4), 20–33.

Mitchell, D. (1998) The origins of learning disability nursing. *International History of Nursing Journal*, **4**(1), 10–16.

Mitchell, D. (2000) Parallel stigma? Nurses and people with learning disabilities. *British Journal of Learning Disabilities*, **28**(2), 78–81.

Mitchell, D. (2003) Threat of the generic nurse. *Learning Disability Practice*, **6**(2), 34.

Navrady, E. (1998) Challenging behaviour: Peplau's model of nursing. *Learning Disability Practice*, **1**(2), 18–21.

Philpot, T. (1995) What the papers say: media images of people with learning difficulties. In Philpot, T. and Ward, L. (eds) *Values and Visions: Changing Ideas in Services for People with Learning Difficulties*. Butterworth Heinemann, Oxford.

Raynes, N.V., Wright, K., Shiell, A. & Pettipher, C. (1994) *The Cost and Quality of Community Residential Care*. David Fulton Publishers, London.

Richardson, M. (1997) Reflection and celebration – Neal (1960–87): narrative of a young man with profound and multiple disabilities. *Journal of Learning Disabilities for Nursing, Health and Social Care*, **1**(4), 191–5.

Ryan, J. & Thomas, F. (1980) *The Politics of Mental Handicap*. Penguin, Harmondsworth.

Scott, C. (1998) Specialist practice: advancing the profession? *Journal of Advanced Nursing*, **28**(3), 554–62.

Southon, G. & Braithwaite, J. (1998) The end of professionalism? *Social Science and Medicine*, **46**(1), 23–8.

Spencer, P. (2002) Support system. *Learning Disability Practice*, **5**(7), 16–20.

Turnbull, J. (1997) Learning disability nursing: a position paper. *Journal of Learning Disabilities for Nursing, Health and Social Care*, **1**(4), 186–90.

Turnbull, J. (2002) Old habits. *Learning Disability Practice*, **5**(7), 3.

Turnbull, J. & Timblick, D. (1998) Residential care homes: the challenge. *Learning Disability Practice*, **1**(2), 10–13.

Woods, P.L. (1997) Conceptualizing advanced nursing practice: curriculum issues to consider in the educational preparation of advanced nurses in the UK. *Journal of Advanced Nursing*, **25**(4), 820–28.

Chapter 2

Getting the balance right: the issues of rights and responsibilities in learning disability

Tim Riding

Down but not out

After being made redundant twice by the age of 20, I was beginning to question the wisdom of my decision to pursue a career in engineering. Whilst contemplating the options open to me, my memory returned to an outward bound course I attended in the first year of my apprenticeship. During the course, we had been asked to develop and host a two-day entertainment programme for a group of children with learning disabilities who were staying at a nearby campsite.

The first day was a great success. However, that evening, one of the youngsters, a 14 year-old girl called Tracy with diabetes and something called 'challenging behaviour', decided to seek out her own entertainment. She left the campsite unaccompanied and wandered off alone. Not such a problem, you'd be forgiven for thinking, if it hadn't been for the fact that she'd wandered off across country into the heart of the Brecon Beacons, with night falling and without her next dose of insulin.

In conjunction with the local constabulary, a delegation was quickly mobilised in a military style manoeuvre to track Tracy down and return her to camp. After several hours of combing the countryside we returned to base to report our lack of success, only to learn that Tracy had been sighted in a nearby village. We ventured out once again and, after several further hours of searching, we stumbled across the cold and terrified 14 year-old huddled in the doorway of the local post office. To my amazement Tracy refused point blank to come back with us and didn't appear the least bit concerned that her injection was now well overdue. After reasoning with her for what seemed like an eternity, Tracy eventually gave in and the day drew to a satisfactory conclusion.

Now, with all the tools of a reflective practitioner, not to mention the benefit of hindsight, it is easy to see why this experience had such an impact on me. It had certainly fulfilled a number of important needs. I was acting in a good cause, possibly saving someone's life. This was not something that just anyone could do and there was a degree of personal risk involved. It was something different and not the sort of thing you did every day of the week. It was also both intriguing and enlightening; at first wondering why someone would behave in such a seemingly *irrational* way, but then understanding how circumstances out of your control can drive you to despair.

A new start

As I arrived home from work with my second redundancy notice in hand, I opened with great anticipation a letter I received that morning from the local psychiatric hospital that said '... further to your recent interview, I have great pleasure in offering you the position of nursing assistant.' I commenced work there some three weeks later and, after cutting my teeth for nearly a year, entered student nurse training aspiring to the status of Registered Nurse of the Mentally Handicapped, as it was called then. The training was both demanding and rewarding and there were many parallels to be drawn with my earlier experience. Then, after three years hard labour, brimming with newly found knowledge and confidence, I set foot on the wards as a qualified nurse, only to be told that I could now learn how to do the job properly.

Working at a secure hospital, the emphasis was on maintaining a secure environment and not necessarily on nursing. Indeed, the latter was often seen as getting in the way of the former. There were a number of very strong role models to learn from; they were not always positive but strong, nevertheless. As the months passed I grew accustomed to the rites and rituals that were characteristic of the setting. Many of them made good sense, though it also occurred to me that some of the skills I acquired during training were seldom practised, and the two were not mutually exclusive. The early years were therefore interspersed by attempts to improve standards of nursing by using nursing models, assessment protocols and systems of care coordination, to name but a few.

Following three unsuccessful attempts to develop my career via a secondment for RMN training, probably the best thing that ever happened to me, I opted for a more academic route instead. I first completed a Diploma in Health Studies and then a degree. I found an increasing range of opportunities available to me, initially as a team leader and then as a clinical leader. It was at that time I was subject to perhaps the greatest influence of my career to date. Working under the auspices of one of the authors of *Continuing the Commitment* (Kay *et al.*, 1995) I found myself in the midst of a revitalised and rejuvenated team, driving through a number of dynamic and innovative changes within the hospital. I discovered that secure care and good nursing were most definitely not mutually exclusive.

A change of direction

On completion of my first degree the executive nurse urged me to undertake a research degree to explore the effectiveness of therapeutic programmes within the hospital for offenders with learning disabilities. In the wake of a damaging inquiry some two years earlier renewed attention on the core business of delivering positive clinical outcomes was a much needed and welcome relief. Given the predominance of sexual offenders within the service, it was subsequently agreed that the focus of the study should centre on that client group. Little did I know it at the time, but as a direct result of that informal conversation I was about to embark on a whole new direction in my career.

The first thing that struck me in the course of the study was 'what therapeutic programme?' Despite an average length of stay of 14 years, none of the clients in question had so far attended a relevant treatment programme. Therefore, working closely with multidisciplinary colleagues, we established a treatment group and decided on the methodology by which we would evaluate it. The plans went almost without hitch and the group settled into its working phase. However, with barely half the programme completed, the decision by commissioners to relocate all high secure learning disability services within England onto a single site, and not the site on which I was currently employed, brought the whole initiative to something of a premature end.

Community bound

I was lucky enough to have acquainted myself with the local community-based learning disability services around that time and didn't hesitate to jump at the position of clinical nurse specialist. Upon my appointment I felt enthused by an overwhelming commitment within the team to serving, and improving the lives of, people with learning disabilities. Person-centred planning was already well established. I was also struck by the complexity of need presented by many of the service users, not only those moving back into the city from secure placements, but those who seemed to be on the fringes of the criminal justice system.

Staff within the directorate were highly motivated and took a dynamic view of the service. Consequently, within a short period of time we had set up a community-based treatment programme for sexual offenders and perpetrators of sexual abuse. A range of other exciting ventures followed, including the development of clinical practice guidelines; clinical effectiveness measures; an assessment tool designed specifically for sexual offenders with learning disabilities; joint risk assessment and management protocols; introduction of the care programme approach and so on. Subsequently, following a successful bid to develop a nurse consultant post, I applied for, and was appointed to the role in March 2000, and took up post that July.

There continues to be a range of influences on my practice. The service in which I work prides itself on the fact that much of the recently published guidance on person-centred planning (Department of Health, 2002) was actually tried and tested here in the north-west. Person-centred planning really does work, even with people with some of the most complex needs. Overall, the NHS Trust has a strong commitment to quality improvement within the framework of clinical governance. There is also a culture of change and innovation, and calculated risk-taking that makes it all the more rewarding to support people like Alan.

Meeting Alan

I first met Alan almost five years ago, when the local health authority referred him to me. An active, almost aggressive policy of resettling people in 'out of area' placements prevailed and, as Alan was a resident in one of the region's medium secure units (MSUs) at the time, funding was therefore to be made available in the next financial year to return him to the community. The proposed model, already yielding great successes with a number of other service users with complex needs, was the supported living model. That is, Alan would enter into a contract with a housing association, or private landlord, as one of their tenants, and a package of individual support would be offered from one of the independent sector provider agencies (Emerson *et al.*, 1998, 1999).

My task, in conjunction with Alan's social worker, was to conduct an assessment of his needs, write the service specification, develop a care plan and risk management plan, assist in the recruitment of Alan's individual staff team, work with the team to ensure they were able to implement relevant aspects of the care plan and risk management plan, deliver relevant aspects of the plan myself and maintain a monitoring and coordinating role under the auspices of the Care Programme Approach (CPA) (Department of Health, 1990; Social Services Inspectorate/NHS Executive, 1998).

On reflection, the decision to bring Alan back to the local area appeared entirely sensible. As Beacock (2001) maintains: 'Empowerment, maximising choice, achieving social integration and promoting independence have been at the top of the shopping list for most users, carers, practitioners and providers for the last 15 years'. However, the challenge, when working with someone with a history of offending, is to strike the right balance between the ideals of Valuing People (Department of Health, 2001a), whilst maintaining both individual and public safety. Consequently, the process of assessment began in earnest.

Despite his tender years, only 23 of them, Alan had what might be described as a colourful and chequered history. He was reported to have made frequent hoax calls to the emergency services, though he had never been charged with these offences. He had also displayed a range of oppositional behaviours, such as putting noxious substances in people's food, running away, verbal abuse, threats of violence and actual physical assault, albeit of a relatively minor nature. Most worryingly, though, was the offence that had led to Alan's admission to the MSU. Some four years earlier he had been charged with the indecent assault of two females. He was remanded to a young-offender institution, and subsequently convicted of the offence and detained under Section 37/41 of the Mental Health Act, 1983.

When I was introduced to Alan he welcomed me with open arms. He thought I was the saviour who was going to take him home and, unsurprisingly, it was easy to strike up a rapport with him. I explained my role, and what I proposed to do by way of assessment. Alan told me he was looking forward to going home with great anticipation, and how he couldn't be bothered with all that nonsense because it was now in the past. Probably not for the first time there was a mismatch between what I, as the professional, wanted to do and Alan, as the recipient of my received wisdom, thought necessary. Therein lay the first challenge to our relationship.

Should I abandon my clinical and professional objectives in the name of choice and rights, or do what I judged needed to be done? I was not about to desert my post that quickly. After all, assessment is described as one of the core skills of the learning disability nurse (Kay *et al.*, 1995). I returned to the purpose of my role, using every ounce of persuasiveness, to try and convince Alan that it was ultimately in his best interests to engage with the assessment process. Moreover, the truth of the matter was that, unless he engaged, his return to the community could actually be jeopardised. However, heeding the cliché that the truth sometimes hurts, and given Alan's history of 'oppositional' behaviour, I thought it wise not to state this too explicitly just yet, for fear of losing his cooperation completely. As Perkins (1991) asserted, praise and persuasion are likely to be needed in equal measure, and at different times, in a more challenging situation. Thankfully, Alan recognised the veracity of my arguments and agreed to what had to be done.

Getting down to planning

The assessment began with the Essential Lifestyle Plan (ELP) (Smull, 1989). This meant asking what were the essential, important and desirable components of Alan's favoured lifestyle. What did a good day look like? What were Alan's strengths and needs? What did he need to keep him healthy and safe? The importance of planning *with* instead of *for* people with learning disabilities has since been recognised in the Department of Health (2002) guidance. The service specification was already beginning to take shape. The risk assessment, and determination of the nature and extent of Alan's needs for continuing clinical interventions, however, out of necessity, proceeded at a slower rate.

As a clinical expert, supporting people with complex needs and offending histories, we are aware that there is a perception amongst the public that we are able to provide a guarantee of no further offending, acting as a magician rather than clinician. Indeed, this view is perpetuated by the frequently asked question 'Will he do it again?' (Prins, 1990). It is important to resist the temptation to offer such assurances. Turner (2000) highlighted the serious limitations in trying to predict future offending and, as Clare (1993) argued, the aim of risk assessment is not to predict recidivism, but to clarify the factors contributing to the aetiology and maintenance of the individual's offending behaviour. Therefore, clinical risk assessments should not be judged by how accurately they predict future offending, but rather as a means of understanding the factors influencing behaviour, and the resultant implications for future behaviour and behaviour change (Litwack *et al.*, 1993).

Kay *et al.* (1995) suggest that only validated schedules should be used during the assessment process. However, the difficulty of conforming to this in relation to offenders with learning disabilities, is that such assessment tools are not readily available or do not even exist (Hames, 1993). Nevertheless, a number of protagonists advocate assessment protocols for risk assessment in general (Turner, 1998, 2000), and sexual offending in particular (see for example, Day, 1997; Murphy, 1997; Thompson & Brown, 1997; O'Connor & Rose, 1998). A local policy and procedure for Joint Risk Assessment and Management Plans (J-RAMP) (Williams *et al.*, 1999) was also under development, and provided further, localised guidance.

Warning signs

Several weeks into the assessment, Alan started to express some rather disturbing views regarding the women he had indecently assaulted. He said that it was all 'their fault', they were 'asking for it' and that he would 'finish the job off' given half the chance. Despite nearly four years in the MSU, a pattern of cognitive distortions consistent with reoffending remained, and Alan had acquired nothing in the way of relapse prevention strategies. The host clinical team defended their position, claiming that Alan was non-compliant with the psychological treatments offered, and had hitherto not presented any management problems. Nevertheless, the decision to resettle Alan in his local community was now open to serious challenge. The second critical juncture was upon us.

A meeting was convened to review the plans. Representatives from the health authority, social services, and host and receiving clinical teams gathered to discuss the options. My position was that I did not feel Alan could be safely supported in a less restrictive setting. He had already absconded on three occasions from the MSU, and now he was telling us that he would reoffend if the opportunity presented itself. How could we possibly hope to manage these risks in a supported living model? Conversely, commissioners, driven by an overriding sense of person-centredness, believed that if the conditions of his ELP could be met, Alan would not be disposed to offending. As I presented the evidence to support my arguments, the weight of opinion gradually shifted in my favour.

The host clinical team acknowledged that alternative strategies could perhaps be employed to encourage Alan to comply with treatment. Commissioners also accepted that if the care package were to be sustained, he would need to complete, or at least start, treatment before leaving the MSU. The decision to support Alan's application for a conditional discharge was thus deferred, and my 'villain of the piece' complex slowly began to dissipate. Other than for subsequent discussions with counterparts at the MSU, and attendance at periodic CPA reviews, my direct involvement with Alan was held in abeyance. Nevertheless, it came as no surprise when, almost three years later, I received the long-awaited phone call.

Getting to know Alan again

Alan was nearing the end of a cognitive behavioural therapy group. He had responded extremely well to treatment and was highly motivated to manage his future behaviour. Alan's Mental Health Review Tribunal (MHRT) was drawing nearer, and now, the multidisciplinary team felt able to support his application; could we revive the plans to resettle him? The receiving multidisciplinary team was reconstituted and work to complete the J-RAMP recommenced. Clare & Murphy (1998) suggested that a successful intervention package is likely to comprise three essential elements: lifestyle changes, direct treatment and prevention or management of further offending. The J-RAMP addressed each in its own way.

It was intended that Alan would return to a self-contained flat, in a complex containing a total of six flats. The building was owned by a local housing trust, and residents of the flats were required to enter into tenancy agreements with the trust. The contract to provide social support to the tenants, however, had been awarded to an independent sector provider agency. Each tenant would receive a specified number of hours of individual support, and access to a core team at other times. Alan was deemed to require 105 hours of individual support per week, at least initially, the primary aim being to promote his access to a range of social, recreational and vocational opportunities, in line with his accomplishments (O'Brien, 1987).

Direct treatment consisted of a continuation of the work already started in the MSU. Clearly this had already had an impact, although Alan's relapse prevention plan indicated the need for ongoing support to help him identify and challenge (re)emerging cognitions consistent with offending behaviour. Using a cognitive behavioural approach (Turnbull, 2000), the sessions were to be held every two weeks, and would focus on Alan's daily recordings in an audio-diary. The aim was to help him establish the link between cognitions and behaviour, and then, using 'Socratic' questioning techniques (Lindsay *et al.*, 1998) to help him arrive at an alternative and incompatible conception. A contract detailing the frequency and conduct of sessions, and clearly highlighting the limits of confidentiality was developed, and Alan's informed consent was sought (Clare & Murphy, 1998).

In addition, the likelihood of further offending was to be reduced by careful monitoring of Alan's behaviour and mental state. Functional analysis (Cullen, 1993; Emerson, 1995) had identified two predominant setting conditions for offending behaviour: low mood and subsequent misuse of alcohol. It was, therefore, proposed that in addition to a daily journal, the Bech-Rafaelsen Melancholia Scale (MES) would also be completed on a weekly basis. Although Alan was not formally diagnosed with a depressive illness, nine of the MES's eleven items specifically related to behaviours he was known to exhibit, suggesting that he was entering a 'sub clinical' depressive episode. As such it was hoped that the MES would provide an early warning system, that would in turn allow for the deployment of reactive risk management strategies.

As envisaged, the MHRT duly granted Alan's conditional discharge under section 73 of the Mental Health Act, 1983. Some six weeks later, with final preparations in place, the transition from secure to community care was effected. Despite his initial apprehension, and one or two teething problems, the move was quite unremarkable. The schedule of appointments and meetings laid out within the J-RAMP was put into practice and all appeared well. That was of course until the voices of dissent began to emerge: there was a problem with the MES.

Alan objected to having to complete the scale on a weekly basis. It was something he viewed as the province of hospitals and psychiatrists; something Alan thought he had left behind. The direct care staff, probably feeding on Alan's disquiet, also began to voice their objections. Didn't they know Alan well enough to 'sense' when he was low? Should they really be asking him to do something against his will? And couldn't it therefore actually have a negative impact on him? This was yet another critical point in my relationship with Alan. It raised a host of issues in relation to his capacity to consent, his legal status and the implications of his refusal to cooperate. It was also a direct threat to my perceived authority and accountability for the discharge of my responsibilities.

Decisive moments

My first sensible thought was not to get drawn into an argument, but to take a step back and carefully weigh the issues. Alan was still, in effect, a detained patient under the jurisdiction of the Home Office. Non-compliance with any aspect of his care plan could lead to recall. To use this as a threat, however, would almost certainly undermine, if not destroy, our relationship. Conversely, the prospect of being hauled in front of an inquiry for failing to prevent the commission of a predictable offence was an equally unattractive proposition. As such, two options began to loom. First, was there an alternative, valid and reliable method to monitor Alan's mood? Or, second, could further steps be taken to gain his compliance?

On reflection, the latter was probably an area I had neglected in my verve to have the J-RAMP sanctioned. Nonetheless, the importance of maximising the role of all team members in the planning and delivery of care is well recognised (Sines & Barr, 1998; Weinstein, 1998), hence the former question was posed: could anyone propose an equally valid and reliable method for monitoring Alan's mood? Only in the subsequent absence of any practical suggestions did I then turn my attention to convincing Alan of the veracity and integrity of my rationale for use of the MES.

Although predating the recently published guidance on seeking consent from people with learning disabilities (Department of Health, 2001b), based on what was already recognised as good practice, I set about providing Alan with enough information in a form that was readily accessible to him, to satisfy myself that his current reluctance was truly informed. The anticipated benefits of carrying out the assessment were reiterated. The lack of suitable alternatives and the risks of not monitoring were explored. And finally, some pragmatic suggestions as to how any 'nuisance effect' could be minimised were put forward. The discussion took place in private at Alan's request, though he was then given a week to discuss the issues with whoever he chose – family, paid carers, even staff back at the hospital.

During my next visit Alan informed me of his decision to comply with the monitoring process. Whilst breathing a sigh of relief, I also thought it important to reflect on what had taken place. Alan was a strong-minded individual with firm views on things affecting his life. He was not always immediately forthcoming with his views, however, and I would need to afford more effort to eliciting them in future. I hoped that both Alan and his care workers had learnt that although at times my interventions seemed to be wrapped up in sophisticated clinical jargon, my intentions were good and I ultimately had Alan's best interests at heart. For my part, I had certainly learnt that simply forging ahead, and failing to explain the rationale and win support for my intervention, had the potential to derail the whole package of care.

The next 12 months passed uneventfully. Alan responded well to continuing therapeutic intervention, and his risk management plan was gradually relaxed as he demonstrated an increasing independence. Monitoring of Alan's mood was also discontinued, with the full agreement of all concerned, as he settled into his new lifestyle with growing confidence and self-esteem, and care workers became more accustomed to his ways. In fact, Alan's progress was so remarkable that it soon came to the point where we had to consider the next step in his rehabilitation – moving to his own flat away from the complex in which he currently resided. Although this brought with it the risks associated with letting go, calculated risk-taking was essential to Alan's personal growth (Saunders, 1998) and intrinsic to the pursuit of his accomplishments (O'Brien, 1987).

Temptations

Unfortunately, the search for an appropriate property soon proved to be a more difficult task than at first assumed, with waiting lists of at least six months for all the major housing trusts. It was during this stagnant period that Alan began to draw increasingly on his newly developed social networks to bolster his mood and self-esteem. Whilst the networks were seen as an extremely positive development in cementing Alan's status as a member of the community (Kay, 1993), his use of them was beginning to give cause for concern. Alan had stretched the three nights per week he visited the local pub to five or even six. He was going out earlier, coming home later and the activities that had previously been the focus, such as crib, darts and pool were now secondary to the intoxicating effects of alcohol.

The fact that Alan's drinking had become a problem came as a surprise. Although the vulnerability of people with learning disabilities to such social pressures is recognised (McCusker *et al.*, 1993), Alan had successfully completed an alcohol awareness course (Forbat, 1999) whilst resident in the MSU. Notwithstanding the knowledge he derived from the course, and his earlier exercise of moderation, Alan's quality of life was now suffering. His appearance had become somewhat dishevelled, and he resented any advice, no matter how subtly or tactfully given. Alan had also started to neglect the upkeep of his flat, his diet was poor and, most worryingly of all, his mental health was deteriorating. Furthermore, although attributed to other factors, Alan had also resigned from the part-time job he secured shortly after his discharge from the MSU.

Time to act

Alarm bells were ringing. All the setting conditions that had preceded his offence were in place once again and it was incumbent upon us to act. A range of practical suggestions were put to Alan as to how to control his behaviour. Could he go out later? Could he take less money out with him? Could he stick to agreed times to come home? Could he learn how to politely decline offers of drinks? We also reiterated information in relation to sensible drinking. Based on lessons learnt from the previous critical point in Alan's care, it was imperative that his views on our current intervention were sought, as illustrated from the following excerpt of conversation:

> *Me:* So Alan, do you think these suggestions will help you to control your drinking?
> *Alan:* Not really, no.
> *Me:* Why's that?
> *Alan:* Well, I haven't really got a problem. Well, I have and I haven't.

Me: You've lost me now.

Alan: Well *I* don't think it's a problem, but it is because *you* think it's a problem.

It quickly became apparent that considerable effort would be needed in helping to raise Alan's awareness of how misuse of alcohol could become a problem, and thus increase his motivation. Nonetheless, the single most important lesson for me throughout the time I had known Alan was that he did not like to be told what to do. No matter how accurate, or how virtuous the message, Alan was only likely to heed it if he was allowed to arrive at the conclusion himself. Instinct told me that Alan would rather choose a return to the MSU, with his destiny in a sense in his own hands, than comply with a care plan in which he saw no reason. The type of therapeutic intervention most suited to Alan's needs was also likely to be ineffective if his motivation remained poor (Farrington & Telford, 1996; Forbat, 1999).

Once again, the use of Socratic techniques as described by Lindsay *et al.* (1998) were of invaluable benefit. The areas that had potential to develop into problems were put to Alan, and his views elicited. Where they diverged from societal norms, or Home Office expectations, arguments to the contrary were presented, though in a questioning rather than lecturing manner. In so doing, Alan was enabled to reflect on the possible negative consequences of his behaviour without them being used as a threat against him. He was then able to make an informed choice regarding his future behaviour, as opposed to feeling coerced. Over the course of the next few weeks Alan did exactly that.

Drawing on techniques of 'relapse prevention' (Marlatt & Gordon, 1985), Alan began to recognise a pattern of feelings and thoughts that typically led to his over indulgence. Much of the work had already been done on correcting his 'thinking errors' and Alan now recognised the importance of maintaining control. However, he was still susceptible to social pressure, and so put into practice the strategies suggested at an earlier stage, although this time with a renewed vigour and corresponding degree of success. With a move to his own flat back on track, and ever more imminent, Alan requested, though, that his search for alternative employment be put on hold whilst final preparations for the move be made. In recognition of his efforts, the care team acceded to Alan's request.

In due course, the flat for which Alan had been waiting became vacant, and set in motion a chain of events. The transitional risk management plan that would govern support and supervision levels under the new arrangements was submitted to the local joint investment group. This, together with reports from the multidisciplinary team, was submitted to the Home Office for their approval and Alan and his care staff attended to the logistical concerns common in any house move. Some three weeks later, with the 't's crossed and the 'i's dotted, Alan moved into his new flat on the outskirts of the city centre.

Getting the balance right

In determining the support levels for the transitional risk management plan, there was an interesting paradox that had to be considered. During Alan's progression through the system of secure services it had become apparent that the anticipation and anxiety caused by any move, no matter how positive, was extremely unsettling for him. This often resulted in behavioural manifestations – social withdrawal, verbal aggression, psychosomatic complaints and a general reduction in his levels of motivation. In the past, increased support had been deployed to counteract any problems. Yet the more support deployed, the less Alan actually wanted. Therefore, whereas the multidisciplinary team wished to increase levels of support, at least for the initial period, Alan actually wanted less.

Again, various members of the team were at pains to convince Alan of the benefits of transitional support arrangements, pointing out their temporary nature. It is difficult to establish precisely the extent to which continuing Home Office involvement influenced Alan's decision. Nevertheless, after weighing up his options over several days, Alan eventually signalled his agreement. In recognition of his willingness to compromise, plans for a reduction in support hours were immediately drawn up, describing alternative mechanisms to ensure Alan's safety. Consequently, after the first month had elapsed, sleep-in staff were withdrawn as agreed, and Alan began checking in with staff back at the complex: in person each morning, and by telephone each night.

This was yet another example of the patience and flexibility required to support someone who has offended in the community. We had always sought to promote Alan's choice, independence and inclusion (Department of Health, 2001a), yet constantly had to balance his rights with the requirements of the Mental Health Act 1983 and wider public safety (Clare & Murphy, 1998). Indeed, as Alan grew in confidence and social mobility, his resentment of a conditional discharge became increasingly apparent, so much so that, after a mere two months in his new flat, Alan found himself in front of a Mental Health Review Tribunal (MHRT) seeking an absolute discharge.

The weeks preceding the MHRT were also characterised by an apparent conflict of loyalties. Whilst all those involved in supporting Alan during the last three years were amazed by his progress, we recognised that he was still undergoing a period of great change. My advice to Alan was that the team could not at that point support his application, and that he should consider deferring the MHRT until a sustained period of stability within his flat had been achieved. I did point out, nonetheless, that this was merely the 'professional' view, and urged him to seek the views of his advocate. An invite to Alan's next review meeting was duly extended to his legal advocate so we could explore the issues in a mature and unbiased fashion.

Unfortunately the legal advocate seemed to adopt something of an adversarial approach and declined the invitation. The MHRT went ahead, and as expected Alan's application for absolute discharge was rejected. And that brought us to 2003. Alan was still in his flat, consolidating on the progress made. His consumption of alcohol was (usually) within safe limits, and he continued to enjoy extensive social networks and support. Direct treatment for his offending behaviour was drawn to a satisfactory conclusion and Alan's support hours were reduced from 105 per week to only 20. The one remaining obstacle was his reluctance, or inability, to find employment, which it was believed would provide the necessary lifestyle change (Clare & Murphy, 1998) for a further reduction in support hours, and multidisciplinary support for his second application for absolute discharge.

Conclusion

Although working with an individual who has offended sometimes feels like an isolated and solitary activity, the importance of teamwork cannot be overstated. As a nurse I was responsible for certain important aspects of Alan's overall care. Yet there was a whole array of other team members each with their own essential part to play: the social worker, the psychiatrist, and not least, Alan's direct care workers. Indeed, without the planned and coordinated input of all, it quite simply would not have been possible to *manage* the risks presented, let alone promote such positive and calculated *risk taking*.

As for supporting Alan himself, this has proved to be both a rewarding and challenging experience. At different times it has called upon a range of different skills: assessment, coordination, therapeutic intervention and knowledge of mental health legislation. The more human skills of patience, respect, negotiation and compromise have been required as well, in no small measure. The critical points in my relationship with Alan have also provided a range of opportunities for learning; both about myself and about the clients whom I support. Never underestimate the potential for coercion, perceived or actual, when people are subject to legal sanction. Never assume that people don't have a view merely because they haven't expressed it. Never assume cooperation and willingness because of a lack of dissent. Accept challenges to your authority as a reminder that you are part of a team. And finally, remember, if at first you don't succeed, the likelihood is that one of these important concerns has been overlooked.

References

Beacock, C. (2001) Counting the cost. *Learning Disability Practice*, **4**(3), 5.

Churchill, J. (1998) The independent sector. In: Thompson, T. & Mathias, P. (eds) *Standards and Learning Disability* 2nd edition. Baillière Tindall, London.

Clare, I.C.H. (1993) Issues in the assessment and treatment of male sex offenders with mild learning disabilities. *Sexual and Marital Therapy*, **8**(2), 167–80.

Clare, I.C.H. & Murphy, G.H. (1998) Working with offenders or alleged offenders with intellectual disabilities. In: Emerson, E., Hatton, C., Bromley, J. & Caine, A. (eds) *Clinical Psychology and People with Intellectual Disabilities*. John Wiley & Sons, Chichester.

Cullen, C. (1993) The treatment of people with learning disabilities who offend. In: Howells, K. & Hollin, C.R. (eds) *Clinical Approaches to the Mentally Disordered Offender*. John Wiley & Sons, Chichester.

Day, K. (1997) Sex offenders with learning disabilities. In: Read, S.G. (ed.) *Psychiatry in Learning Disability*. Saunders, London.

Department of Health (1990) *Joint Health and Social Services Circular: The Care Programme Approach for People with a Mental Illness Referred to Specialist Psychiatric Services. HC(90)23/LASSL(90)11.* Department of Health, London.

Department of Health (2001a) *Valuing People: A New Strategy for Learning Disability for the 21st Century*. Department of Health, London.

Department of Health (2001b) *Seeking Consent: Working with People with Learning Disabilities*. Department of Health, London.

Department of Health (2002) *Valuing People: A New Strategy for Learning Disability for the 21st Century. Planning With People. Towards Person Centred Approaches: Guidance for Implementation Groups*. Department of Health, London.

Emerson, E. (1995) *Challenging Behaviour: Analysis and Intervention in People with Learning Difficulties*. Cambridge University Press, Cambridge.

Emerson, E., Robertson, J., Gregory, N., Hatton, C., Kessissoglou, S., Hallam, A., Knapp, M., Järbrink, K., Netten, A., Walsh, P., Linehan, C., Hillery, J. & Durkan, J. (1998) *Quality and Costs of Residential Supports for People With Learning Disabilities: A Comparative Analysis of Quality and Costs in Village Communities, Residential Campuses and Dispersed Housing Schemes*. Hester Adrian Research Centre, Manchester.

Emerson, E., Robertson, J., Gregory, N., Hatton, C., Kessissoglou, S., Hallam, A., Knapp, M., Järbrink, K. & Netten, A. (1999) *Quality and Costs of Residential Supports for People With Learning Disabilities: A Comparative Analysis of Quality and Costs in Group Homes and Supported Living Schemes*. Hester Adrian Research Centre, Manchester.

Farrington, A. & Telford, A. (1996) Naming the problem: assessment and formulation. In: Marshall, S. & Turnbull, J. (eds) *Cognitive Behaviour Therapy: An Introduction to Theory and Practice*. Ballière Tindall, London.

Forbat, L. (1999) Developing an alcohol awareness course for clients with a learning disability. *British Journal of Learning Disabilities*, **27**, 16–19.

Hames, A. (1993) People with learning disabilities who commit sexual offences – assessment and treatment, *NAPSAC Newsletter*, **6**, 3–6.

Kay, A. (1993) Helping with social issues. In: Shanley, E. & Starrs, T.A. (eds) *Learning Disabilities: A Handbook of Care*. Churchill Livingstone, Edinburgh.

Kay, B., Rose, S. & Turnbull, J. (1995) *Continuing the Commitment: The Report of the Learning Disability Nursing Project*. Department of Health, London.

Lindsay, W.R., Neilson, C.Q., Morrison, F. & Smith, A.H.W. (1998) The treatment of six men with a learning disability convicted of sex offences with children. *British Journal of Clinical Psychology*, **37**, 83–98.

Litwack, T.R., Kirschner, S.M. & Wack, R.C. (1993) The assessment of dangerousness and predictions of violence: recent research and future prospects. *Psychiatric Quarterly*, **64**(3), 245–73.

Marlatt, G.A. & Gordon, J. (1985) *Relapse Prevention*. Guilford Press, New York.

McClusker, C.G., Clare, I.C.H., Cullen, C. & Reep, J. (1993) Alcohol-related knowledge and attitudes in people with a mild learning disability: the effects of a 'sensible drinking' group. *Journal of Community and Applied Social Psychology*, **3**, 29–40.

Murphy, G. (1997) Assessing risk. In: Churchill, J., Brown, H., Craft, A. & Horrocks, C. (eds) *There are no easy answers: the provision of continuing care to adults with learning disabilities who sexually abuse others*. ARC, Chesterfield.

O'Brien, J. (1987) A guide to lifestyle planning: using the Activities Catalogue to integrate services and natural support systems. In: Wilcox, B.W. & Bellamy, G.T. (eds) *The Activities Catalogue: An Alternative Curriculum for Youth and Adults with Severe Disabilities*. P.H. Brookes, Baltimore.

O'Connor, C.R. & Rose, J. (1998) Sexual offending and abuse perpetrated with men with learning disabilities: an integration of current research concerning assessment and treatment. *Journal of Learning Disabilities for Nursing, Health and Social Care*, **2**(1), 31–8.

Perkins, D. (1991) Clinical work with sex offenders in secure settings. In: Hollin, C.R. & Howells, K. (eds) *Clinical Approaches to Sex Offenders and Their Victims*. Wiley, Chichester.

Prins, H. (1990) *Dangerousness: A Review of Principle and Practice in Forensic Psychiatry*. Churchill Livingstone, London.

Saunders, M. (1998) Risk management. In: Thompson, T. & Mathias, P. (eds) *Standards and learning disability*, 2nd edition. Baillière Tindall, London.

Sines, D. & Barr, O. (1998) Professions in teams. In: Thompson, T. & Mathias, P. (eds) *Standards and Learning Disability*, 2nd edition. Baillière Tindall, London.

Smull, M.W. (1989) *Crisis in the Community*. National Association of Mental Retardation Program Directors Inc., Virginia.

Social Services Inspectorate/NHS Executive (1998) *Effective Care Coordination in Mental Health Services: Modernising the Care Programme Approach*. Department of Health, London.

Thompson, D. & Brown, H. (1997) Men with intellectual disabilities who sexually abuse: a review of the literature. *Journal of Applied Research in Intellectual Disabilities*, **10**(2), 140–58.

Turnbull, J (2000) Cognitive behavioural interventions. In: Gates, B., Gear, J. & Wray, J. (eds) *Behavioural Distress: Concepts and Strategies*. Baillière Tindall, Edinburgh.

Turner, S. (1998) *The Assessment of Risk and Dangerousness as Applied to People with Learning Disabilities Considered at Risk of Offending. Part 1: Literature Review*. Hester Adrian Research Centre, Manchester.

Turner, S. (2000) Forensic risk assessment in intellectual disabilities: the evidence base and current practice in one English region. *Journal of Applied Research in Intellectual Disabilities*, **13**, 239–55.

Weinstein, J. (1998) The professions and their interrelationships. In: Thompson, T. & Mathias, P. (eds) *Standards and Learning Disability*, 2nd edition. Baillière Tindall, London.

Williams, J., Ferns, C. & Riding, T. (1999) *Policy and Procedure: Joint Risk Assessment and Management (J-RAMP) for Adults with Learning Disabilities*. Liverpool Health Authority, Liverpool Social Services Directorate and North Mersey Community NHS Trust, Learning Disabilities Directorate, Liverpool.

Chapter 3

A partnership for health: respecting choice as part of a healthy lifestyle

Jill Turner

Beginnings

In 1994, I qualified as a registered nurse in learning disabilities. I joined the staff of a National Health Service trust in Oxfordshire as an associate nurse for adults who have a learning disability. During my time with the trust I took the opportunity to progress from associate nurse to manager in a residential setting, then to senior community nurse as part of a specialist community team and, finally, to lecturer practitioner and clinical nurse specialist.

My introduction to nursing is a complex matter. To this day I still wonder what it might have been like if I had followed my original career pathway. As a child I was always inquisitive, wanting to know how things worked and why. I had always dreamed of becoming a mechanical engineer. I always was, and still am, a practical person. My ambition led me to become the victim of age discrimination at 18 years when I was considered too old for the Youth Training Scheme apprenticeships. Dazed and bitter from my experiences I flitted from temporary to permanent posts in offices, shops and warehouses but never really considered any of these as a career. I wanted something I could get into and enjoy: a job where I could look forward to getting up in the morning and facing each new challenge. For some reason, this proved illusive.

A set of horrific circumstances in October 1989 propelled me into the nursing arena. I was knocked down while walking across a zebra crossing and received head injuries and a fractured femur. I was a patient at my local orthopaedic hospital and became the 'difficult patient', taking the opportunity to observe nursing practice and question the nurses and students at every opportunity. When I was discharged some six months later I returned home for a period of convalescence. I completely forgot about nursing, before returning to my previous employment in retail.

During the early months of 1991 the local school of nursing put up a display in the local shopping centre, trying to recruit people into nursing on the new Project 2000 programme. I made enquiries and considered applying for learning disability nursing. So, why did I choose learning disability nursing and not another branch of nursing? At that time I did not know which branch of nursing I specifically wanted to pursue. However, I decided which branch I did not want to pursue, which was adult nursing. I acknowledge that my experience was limited by my time as a patient but I just did not consider it the choice for me. As an inpatient, my observation of hospital nursing was one of continual internal rotation. Nurses never spent more than six months in any one ward. Patients changed almost on a daily basis and just when you remembered one person's name they were gone. As a patient, I felt part of a production line where people came in broken and went out mended. Despite my inquisitive ways, the nurses almost seemed pleased to see me if they had been off duty for more than three days as I was usually the only patient they recognised.

I did not want to work in this type of environment with limited opportunity to get to know people. I wanted a career where I could challenge and be challenged and where I could learn and ask why. I wanted to have a career where I could develop long-term relationships within professional boundaries, where I could get to know people as people and they could get to know me, where I could build a career on trust and mutual respect and where I could feel valued. At that time, my experience of people who have learning disabilities was extremely limited. One previous experience was limited to a summer play scheme with adolescents who had a learning disability, where I have strong memories of having a fantastic time playing. As a child this was one of my favourite summer holidays. As an adult I became more aware of people who have learning disabilities through work placements in the high-street retailer where I was working as a warehouse stock controller. During conversations with the work experience staff during tea breaks I began to realise how different our expectations, choices, life opportunities and experiences were, despite them being the same age as me. I began to realise that people with learning disabilities did not have a visible presence within the local community and perhaps this made it all the more intriguing for me to find out more. This made me determined to pursue a career in learning disability nursing.

In my relatively brief career in learning disability nursing I have been privileged to get to know a few people really well, to share the joy of a smile, the reward of being trusted with personal confidences, of being introduced as 'my friend', providing support to develop health and fight ill health and being permitted to share the experience of mourning the death of a loved one. I value human life highly and the individual contribution we make to humankind and our continual learning and development.

One particularly challenging experience involved discussions between a general practitioner and a parent where I supported the parent. The purpose of the meeting was to discuss the replacement of a gastrostomy tube in order to enable the son to continue to receive fluid and nutrition. The context of the discussion focused on the GP expressing his belief that the adult son, who had a profound learning disability, had no quality of life and had outlived all expectations. The GP had not budgeted for the replacement of the gastrostomy device. This encounter challenged my role in supporting the parent to advocate on their son's behalf for continuing interventions. It reaffirmed my belief that we all have different life experiences and develop our own opinions as to the quality of the lives of others.

Reflecting on my time as a patient attached to traction, month after month and pitying myself, I recalled a conversation with a visitor who had a friend in the spinal injuries unit. The friend had been injured and had also been on traction, and had expressed the view that life wasn't worth living as a paraplegic. We both mourned what we had lost and were frightened of what we were to become. Others would place little value on our respective quality of life but we were both determined to succeed. Our experiences have shaped and changed the manner in which we measure quality and value in our lives.

In my practice situation, the parent valued the son for who he was and not for what he could contribute to society. The GP devalued the son for his use of health resources and the financial cost that could, arguably, be better spent on other patients. I am pleased and relieved to say that, on this occasion, the value of human life prevailed and the son received his replacement gastrostomy device.

Learning from experience

Practice experience is recognised as a rich source of learning (Atkins & Murphy, 1994). However, experience alone is not enough. Reflection is one of many tools that I use as a practitioner to develop my learning experience. Boud *et al.* (1985) and Johns (1994) identified reflection as a conscious process that requires the learner to focus upon a particular event experienced during practice, and explores the experience to establish new understanding and appreciation. Therefore, using the model of reflection devised by Johns (1994), I will reflect upon my role and practice in working with Sue, a woman with learning disabilities.

The English National Board for Nursing, Midwifery and Health Visiting (1985) identified that an initial assessment provides an indication of a person's current level of skills and identifies areas that may then be assessed in greater depth. Initial assessments identified that Sue had several significant areas of unmet need. The area that I will address in this chapter is continence.

My assessment was made through observation and questioning, the use of a continence assessment form, and a selection of frequency and volume baseline recording forms. Following this, a plan of care was addressed and formulated. The way in which care is implemented has implications for its success. Clarke (1991) emphasised the importance that continuity plays within successful provision of care. This will be discussed later when I explain my work with Sue. Consideration will also be given to how nursing intervention can be most effectively implemented. The final, and ongoing stage of the nursing process is the evaluation stage (Kratz, 1979). This stage enables the care to be revised in order to meet the changing needs of the individual. I will use a model of reflection to evaluate the care I planned and implemented (Johns, 1994). From experience I find it beneficial to document the evaluation, as I find it is easier to make a comparison with the established baseline observations and this assists with the measurement of any progress.

Personal history

Sue was a woman who appeared to be an anxious person, apparently lacking confidence and self-esteem. She required intensive support and praise for her achievements. She had a moderate learning disability, the cause of which had never been determined, that was comparable with an intelligence quotient score of 50 or less (Grossman, 1983).

Sue was the youngest of five children, with three sisters and one brother and was the only child living in her parents' home. She attended a special school where she was reported to be coping with her menstruation and personal hygiene. While attending further education the teachers reported that Sue's hygiene 'could be cleaner', that her 'self-help skills were limited' and that Sue 'could be helped by a slightly more supportive home background'. At no time during her education was Sue reported to experience difficulties maintaining her continence.

Involvement from nurses within the community team for people who have a learning disability (CTPLD) commenced with a referral from the school when Sue was 17 years old. The referral requested an assessment of her bathing skills. She was having a bath at school. The school reported that they were also unofficially laundering her clothes. The outcome of the assessment was that Sue was physically independent and was able to bath herself. The intervention that was planned to enable Sue to transfer her bathing skills to the home was short-lived because it was reported that her mother was a poor role model and did not support the nursing intervention.

Other CTPLD professionals became involved with Sue when she was 25 years old. Periodically, during adulthood, Sue required support from a psychologist to enable her to manage her anxieties. However, CTPLD involvement had previously been short-lived because of the complex family dynamics. Discussions with Sue's mother identified a financial reason for her remaining at home with her parents, as they were partially reliant on Sue's income to subsidise the household expenditure. Sue reported to the CTPLD that her sister 'took money and other things' from her. Sue's mother told me that she couldn't look after herself but I believed that her mother did not acknowledge the skills that Sue had attained. Professionally, my occupational therapy colleagues and I envisaged that Sue would quickly develop many of her independent living skills if she had consistent positive support from both her parents and her existing support network.

During the course of my home visits I often heard Sue's mother use derogatory phrases to describe her daughter, which further undermined Sue's confidence and reinforced her desire to seek positive reinforcement from people outside the family. Unfortunately, from observations made during practice, it would be appropriate to say that Sue's home situation was one of conflict between family members which had a continual detrimental impact upon her anxieties and confidence, and further strengthened her need to seek positive reinforcement from people outside the family home.

Sue frequently requested help to leave home. Attempts by CTPLD and care agencies to support Sue to move from her parents' home had been unsuccessful, with Sue changing her mind and choosing to stay at home. She continued to express the wish to move and live with her fiancé but was frightened to leave her mother at home with her father. She reported that her father was verbally and physically abusive towards her. Sue said he came home drunk and that she was frightened for her own and her mother's safety.

As you can see from this personal history, there were a multitude of factors that had the potential to influence the nurse-client relationship and the success of interventions from outside the family.

Getting to know more about Sue

I became involved in supporting Sue following a referral to the CTPLD's nurses when Sue was 29. The referral identified a request from Sue for help to support her with her health concerns. During the initial assessment I established that there were many health issues which Sue reported that included pain passing urine (dysuria), water on the knee (bursitis), asthma, eczema, acute anxieties regarding sun and skin cancer, anxieties about her teeth, blue hands and feet in the winter and back pain after falling off a chair the previous week.

I discussed these issues with Sue and her GP. Sue reported that she experienced pain in her tummy when passing urine. She reported going to the toilet more than eight times a day, sometimes with 'accidents' when she was incontinent of urine. Sue explained that she drank more than four glasses of water each day with no other variety of fluid intakes. Sue also presented symptoms of urgency and frequency. The investigations that were initiated included urinalysis and a mid-stream urine specimen that confirmed the presence of a urine infection and a diagnosis of dysuria and dyspepsia. The GP prescribed co-amoxiclav suspension, and a liquid antacid for the dyspepsia, which was thought to be the cause of Sue's prolonged history of abdominal pain.

Sue asked me not to discuss her health with her mother but she agreed that I could discuss her needs with her key worker at work. I respected Sue's request but explained to her that it would be difficult to support her to meet her health needs if she did not have her mother's help when she was at home. Sue said that she would tell her mother about the appointments with the doctor. I had concerns whether I would be able to give enough physical assistance to Sue as she would need to take the medication during evenings and weekends when I would not be at work. I was also concerned that Sue would not be able to complete the course of antibiotics as prescribed and subsequently could experience repeated infections (Lehne, 1998). Many researchers have identified issues with patient compliance while self-medicating. Cameron (1996) identified five social and psychological influences on patient compliance that included knowledge and understanding, quality of interaction with the health professional, social isolation and social support, health beliefs and attitudes, and illness and treatment. I thought that many of these issues applied to Sue, which added a greater challenge to our partnership and my attempts to meet Sue's health demands.

In order to try to establish her compliance, I provided a thorough explanation and practical demonstration for self-medicating to both Sue and her key worker. Sue also involved her fiancé, who also self-medicated. Sue's fiancé agreed to support Sue with her medication at the weekend and during the evenings when he saw her. I arranged to make a follow-up visit one week later. Upon evaluation Sue identified that she had only taken one dose of the antacid because she said that she did not like the taste, so she stopped taking it. Sue reported that the pain when passing urine had ceased and that she no longer complained of abdominal pain. The frequency of her micturition also reduced to between two and four times daily while she was at work. She stated that her key worker and fiancé had helped her to remember to take her medicine.

Reflection

Due to the following factors, I experienced particular difficulty supporting Sue to self medicate:

- Sue had difficulties with literacy and numeracy and could not read the directions on her medication.
- Sue demonstrated difficulties retaining verbal information.
- Sue demonstrated difficulties retaining associated meaning to graphical/ pictorial instruction.
- Sue did not want her parents to know about my support role.
- Sue did not want her parents to know she was taking medication.

As a result of Sue's difficulties with literacy and numeracy, as well as her difficulties retaining verbal and graphical instruction, I found the existing arrangement presented problems supporting Sue in a consistent way. Clarke (1991) emphasised the importance of ensuring continuity within care provision. The difficulties of compliance faced by individuals who had poor reading skills were recognised by Hussey & Gilliland (1989) who also acknowledged that a person's perception, vocabulary development and organisation of thought could cause misunderstanding and misinterpretation of instructions.

Another significant difficulty was trying to ensure my involvement with supporting Sue did not require my visiting the family home. At Sue's request, appointments were held at her workplace. However, I considered that the environment was not conducive to providing the privacy we required for discussion of sensitive and potentially embarrassing health issues. Although a room was available in which to meet, there were frequent interruptions. Sue was distressed and embarrassed about her pain and incontinence. Many authors have recognised that urinary incontinence can have a detrimental effect upon a person's quality of life within their social, psychological, occupational, domestic, physical and sexual functioning (Cardozo, 1991; Lewey, 1997; Malone-Lee, 1999).

Professionally, I felt frustrated that Sue's mother had such a powerful influence over Sue's beliefs and activities. However, I valued the parental role, with its leadership and role modelling, especially during the formative years. In Sue's situation, her mother appeared to be over-compensating. For example, her apparent determination to refer to Sue as a child and her continuing to do things for her was limiting the opportunity for her to develop and learn the skills necessary to encourage her independence. Throughout my time with Sue, the absence of family support influenced my decision-making and subsequent actions in planning interventions and developing support strategies for Sue. Cameron (1996) recognised the important role of the patient's family when providing physical and emotional support to meet health needs. It is important to recognise that a negative impact can also be exerted. I visualised my role as one of clarifying information and providing constructive support. This was achieved through collaborative working with other health professionals and Sue's key worker.

Within the confines of the complex relationship between Sue, her family and professional support services, I believed that the planned intervention was appropriate and successful. I believed that Sue was well supported throughout the experience by myself and her key worker, as well as receiving the informal support from her fiancé. Sue was encouraged and supported to participate with her own care. Cameron (1996) recognised patient participation in their care as leading towards increased patient motivation and increased compliance with treatment. Sue's limitations with numeracy and literacy were overcome by the provision of support by her key worker, who encouraged and assisted Sue to self-administer her medication, and additional informal support was provided by her fiancé. This episode of care could have been improved if I had been able to involve Sue's mother from the outset, as Sue would have been supported with her medication during the weekend. Consistency of support could have been improved. However, on this occasion, the medication was a short course, the support provided was adequate and subsequently the infection cleared.

A thriving relationship

Following this experience I felt more comfortable about supporting Sue with health issues and not involving the family in supporting Sue. I built a strong professional relationship with Sue, her key worker and fiancé. I also believed my knowledge and understanding of continence issues increased considerably.

Earlier in this chapter I stated that I value the opportunity to get to know people as people highly. In getting to know Sue, and developing our professional relationship, initially Sue and I established verbal agreement on my role. She referred to me as 'Jill – my community nurse'. She expected me to visit her each week while I completed my assessment. Sue entrusted me with detailed personal information about her family and I, in turn, divulged enough detail about my family to appear open. I kept Sue informed of my actions and the possibility of needing to share this information with my colleagues. I involved Sue in all decisions about her health needs. We held bimonthly review meetings to which Sue invited relevant people. She usually took the lead at these meetings. Throughout our relationship, my perception was that Sue was pleased to have someone she considered to be on her side, to whom she could entrust secrets, and talk about embarrassing things without being made fun of. Sue often described situations, arising from incontinence, where she felt bullied and not liked by her family and so-called friends. Sue recalled many embarrassing episodes of incontinence that limited her social opportunities.

A relationship for health

During the following 18 months I continued to support Sue to maintain and improve both her physical and psychological health. Sue required many more interventions as a result of her complaints of abdominal pain and her urinary incontinence. As my professional relationship with Sue developed she permitted me to meet her mother. During separate discussions with Sue's mother I became increasingly aware that Sue took everything her mother said to be a medical fact. Sue appeared to somatise, although not formally diagnosed by the psychiatrist, when her mother felt unwell. Sue frequently reported to me that she experienced the same symptoms as her mother. Throughout that time Sue said she was going for 'big poos' each day, complained of 'wetting her pants' at work and had intermittent pain in the right-hand side of her abdomen. The GP previously prescribed paracetamol, and then co-proxamol, as required, for analgesia. I was informed that Sue did not request the medication from her family or carers at work. As I explained earlier, Sue had difficulties with literacy and recollection of verbal instruction. Therefore, the medication was ineffective in meeting Sue's needs. This added a greater emphasis on Sue's need for a supporting network amongst her family, employer and fiancé.

Sue previously described that she was fearful that she would have episodes of urinary or faecal incontinence in public. These fears often resulted in Sue choosing not to eat or drink while out, unless a toilet was in close proximity. Even then, Sue might not use the toilet effectively and she explained that they were often dirty or did not contain toilet paper. Sue reported that she was frightened of getting an infection from a dirty toilet. She informed me that her mother had told her not to use dirty toilets. Sue had developed a posture that did not require her to sit on the toilet. Walsh (1997) identified the skill of maintaining appropriate body posture during micturition as a basic skill required for achieving urinary continence.

My observations identified that Sue's posture would present problems if it remained unchanged. I provided pictorial information and demonstration for correct seating position and encouraged Sue to sit on the toilet fully and count to ten to provide an opportunity for her posture to remain in seated position and let nature take its course. Additionally, in an attempt to partially compensate for her fears, I reassured Sue that she could not pick up an infection and encouraged her to purchase a pocket pack of moist toilet tissues so that she would be able to wipe the seat and have tissues available to wipe her self. This appeared to be implemented successfully and was affordable for Sue with her limited budget.

Unfortunately, within 18 months of this intervention, Sue reported that she had been incontinent in her local shopping centre. Sue was again complaining about pain in her abdomen on passing urine. I arranged an appointment with the GP. Sue said that she experienced pain whilst passing urine and stools. The results of a mid-stream urine sample identified an absence of infection. On this occasion I arranged with Sue and her key worker to complete a bladder diary (frequency chart) for seven days.

Following completion of the diary and during discussion with Sue it became apparent that she was experiencing urinary incontinence at work. It was difficult to analyse the information because of the inconsistency in recording. Therefore, I could not determine the exact frequency, but the information suggested a routine of voiding urine between two and five times each day at work. Several days recording identified voiding at hourly intervals. Sue said that she had a sensation of when she needed to go to the toilet but didn't like to use public toilets because of the reasons she had given before. Sue also said that she did not like to use the toilets at work because people disturbed her by knocking on the door.

These factors, in addition to my own observations of Sue's toilet posture while gaining her previous urine sample, gave me reason for concern that she might not be emptying her bladder completely when voiding and could be experiencing residual urine. Getliffe & Dolman (1997) identified the risks of residual urine contributing to developing urine infection and formation of bladder stones or calculi. During a subsequent appointment with Sue's GP an MSU specimen was collected and urinalysis identified absence of infection. On physical examination, a physical cause of the pain could not be identified.

Sue was encouraged to continue taking analgesia as required. A referral was made for an abdominal ultrasound examination, to identify possible renal calculi, and a referral was made to the continence advisory service for ultrasound examination of the bladder to determine whether Sue was experiencing incomplete bladder emptying and subsequent residual urine. The results of both ultrasound examinations reported that nothing abnormal could be detected.

During a discussion with Sue and her key worker, I suggested bladder retraining through posture management, using the toilet at specific intervals and reducing fluid intake to drinking one litre of water at work while continuing usual intake of drinks at home. Cardozo (1991) identified that women who had a high fluid intake when frequency of micturition is a problem should restrict their fluid intake. An additional intervention I considered was teaching pelvic floor exercises. Many authors have asserted the benefits of a well-toned pelvic floor for maintaining bladder and bowel continence (Norton, 1997; Malone-Lee, 1999; Moore & Fader, 1999).

After reading the literature and in discussions with Sue, I established that Sue had difficulties understanding how her body worked. She had found previous vaginal examinations acutely distressing. Due to these sensitivities accurate assessment of pelvic floor function was not possible. In order that pelvic floor muscle rehabilitation is successful Markwell & Sapsford (1998) identified that the patient must have understanding and awareness of what they are doing. I therefore considered that, as a direct result of Sue's difficulties, teaching pelvic floor exercises or the use of electro-stimulation and biofeedback techniques would be inappropriate for Sue at that time.

Because of my previous work with Sue I felt, during assessment, it would be appropriate to use a pictorial chart to aid recognition and identification of stool type (Lewis & Heaton, 1997) rather than verbal description alone. Subsequently, when I asked Sue about 'having a poo', she described that she had 'runny poo'. To provide more detail within the assessment I also asked Sue and her key worker to complete a food and fluid diary and bowel diary for one week. This would provide me with greater detail regarding bowel motility, dietary fibre and fluid intake.

Once again, the detail of recorded information was poor, with much of the information missing or inaccurate. I reviewed the week's diary entries and estimation in collaboration with Sue's key worker, and we identified that Sue was going to the toilet at work, opening her bowels once a day and her stools varied from liquid to hard. In discussion about Sue's diet, it appeared that she had little appetite, saying she felt 'full up', 'was getting fat' and 'was on a diet'. Sue was eating a restricted diet with little or no fruit, vegetables and dietary fibre.

In discussion with Sue and her key worker I provided information on healthy eating with suggestions on including five fruit and vegetable portions a day in line with current dietary recommendations (Department of Health, 1995). In a follow-up appointment Sue stated that she had taken the information leaflet home and her mother had thrown it away. The key worker thought that Sue had the opportunity to change what she ate at work and could buy fruit from the local shop to eat at work. Once again the issues of continuity of care provision and compliance arose.

A further appointment with the GP identified, during abdominal palpation, that Sue had impacted faeces. The GP said that there were stools in both the ascending and transverse colon with an empty rectum. The GP prescribed a short course of senna syrup at night and lactulose solution in the day. Once again I was concerned about Sue's compliance with this regime. Sue agreed that I could discuss her constipation with her mother.

The planned intervention addressed fluid intake, bladder retraining, medication and dietary change. Once the stools became soft and easier to pass Sue stopped taking the medication. Her reason for stopping was partly due to the taste and also due to increased flatulence and soft, sticky stools. Despite my explanation about these effects being all right, and part of the action of the medication, Sue said she did not want any more medication. I continued encouraging Sue and her mother to address the problem through diet and fluid. Sue chose to continue with her food diary for three more weeks. She was encouraged to buy fruit to eat at work and to eat a healthy lunch from the canteen at work.

The interventions completed during this care episode included:

- Mid-stream urine (MSU) specimen and urinalysis, with a positive result requiring antibiotic therapy.
- Pregnancy test to rule out ectopic pregnancy.
- Smear test, vaginal swab and abdominal examination to rule out a genito-urinary infection, specifically pelvic inflammatory disease.
- Ultrasound examination of abdomen to rule out bladder, kidney and gall stones.

A steep learning curve

Several of these investigations were new experiences for me. I had not previously supported someone through consultation for examination for either ectopic pregnancy or ultrasound examination. Therefore, I needed to bring my understanding of procedures up to date while developing wider professional relationships with practitioners in the local general hospital. My role was one of supporting Sue while managing and dispelling some of her anxieties and, at the same time, providing sufficient information to enable her to make an informed choice about her examinations and also the consequences if she chose not to go through with the examinations, without frightening Sue with information overload.

During reflection I began to consider that many of the symptoms Sue had been presenting intermittently during the previous months were probably due to unidentified constipation. Withell (2000) identified the predisposing factors in constipation to be inadequate fibre intake, inhibiting toilet facilities and neurological disorders. With hindsight I realise that had the presenting symptoms been recognised (abdominal pain, distended abdomen, occasional nausea, headaches and anorexia), then dietary intervention could have been initiated earlier. On this occasion I was able to involve Sue's mother who was, on the whole, a positive influence on the success of the intervention at home. Sue's key worker remained a source of positive encouragement and motivation for her at work.

Factors affecting dietary influences on constipation include finances, food and fluid intake, medication, mobility and the individual's ability to shop and cook (Winney, 1998). A detrimental factor was Sue's financial situation. Sue came from an impoverished family that was reliant upon benefits. Sue's mother had limited income to buy fresh foods and the family's preferences for white bread and sugary cereals limited the opportunity for her to make healthier food selections at home. The other important positive factor was the support, once again, from Sue's fiancé. Sue and her fiancé went shopping together each Saturday. He encouraged Sue to buy fruit and healthy snacks to take to work the following week. He also encouraged Sue to select healthier meals in the canteen at work.

Winney (1998) identified that constipation is rarely life threatening and is often seen as little more than an inconvenience which is generally distressing and uncomfortable for the individual who experiences it. With hindsight I identified that, for all involved in assessment and treatment, with greater clarity of interpreting the reported symptoms, the situation could have been better managed and intervention could have been initiated earlier. Earlier intervention would have alleviated some of the symptoms Sue experienced. Having worked through the experience I forged stronger partnerships with members of the local general hospital, primary healthcare team and continence advisory service. Should the situation recur, I would feel better equipped to identify the symptoms to initiate earlier intervention.

A family affair

The main moral and ethical dilemma faced throughout my time working with Sue was that of her home situation. She openly complained about her family and it was obvious to the observer that she lived in impoverished and neglected circumstances. She loved her mother and was frightened to leave her at home with her father when he had been drinking. Sue was frightened of her father when he was drunk but loved him when he was sober. This proved a constant emotional dilemma for Sue. Consequently, she often expressed feeling unsupported by her family. As a health professional I have the support of the health organisations and local statutory and voluntary authorities and through these organisations and authorities I have the opportunity to support people to make decisions to initiate changes in their lives.

However, despite Sue's complaints she chose to remain at home. I am not convinced that Sue was truly able to make an informed choice to stay. This emotive situation played a significant part in her decision-making processes. Sue has had a limited experience of lifestyles to make an informed choice and chose what she felt was safest for her mother. Emotionally I found this dilemma extremely difficult to cope with. I felt uncomfortable and powerless to change anything when faced by Sue in tears on an almost daily basis. I was fortunate to be able to reflect on my situation with my clinical supervisor, which enabled me to offload my personal distress and put my role and responsibilities into perspective. I have been able to continually develop my knowledge and clinical skills via a combination of empirical evidence and informal knowledge.

Compared to the complex needs of many individuals I have had the privilege to work with, in my naivety I thought that the need to regain continence, expressed by Sue, would be reasonably straightforward to achieve through lifestyle changes including modifications to her diet and exercise routines. However, Sue's motivation and commitment alone was insufficient for the goal to be achieved. In practice, it proved to be one of the most challenging groups of needs I have encountered in one case. Throughout my intervention I continually evaluated my role and the fragility of our nurse-client relationship. At all times I was aware of the imbalance of power between us. Sue looked to me for support and guidance when faced with family confrontations. At all times I was aware that I was a guest in the family home and one wrong move could prevent me returning. This was something Sue regularly referred to as her parents had barred team members from supporting her in the past.

Throughout my interventions I continually strived to act in an advocate role (UKCC, 1992) with emphasis on supporting Sue to uphold her rights as an adult who was being disempowered by her family. My attempts to support Sue to take increased control of her health and meet her own needs were frequently thwarted. Sue set her goals against those of her family who maintained their financially and emotionally dominating role throughout my interventions. As a professional I accepted that Sue was making her own life choices. Although these may not achieve optimum physical or psychological health, they were the choices Sue wanted to make.

However, the ultimate need expressed by Sue was to become more independent. Sue identified that she would like someone else to talk to about the difficulties at home and help her to work things out with her family. I arranged an appointment with a local citizen advocacy group. Sue met with the advocate and talked about her difficulties at home but became anxious when conversation turned towards how to address these difficulties. Following several meetings Sue identified that she had changed her mind and didn't want to upset her mother by talking to her about any of her worries about living at home. I became rather frustrated at this point as I could not identify how else to support Sue to improve her circumstances at home and I found it difficult to accept that Sue was freely choosing to live with these difficulties on a daily basis. To fuel my professional frustrations Sue continued to complain about problems at home on a weekly basis and also continued to 'offload' onto her fiancé and her work colleagues.

Several weeks later the employer informed me that they had invited a local self-advocacy group to visit. Sue told me all about the group and how many of her friends were already members. She also told me that they were helping her to say 'No' and make choices about her money and her life. As Sue became more empowered and more self aware, her confidence increased, leading her towards her personal goal of independence. Through joining a self-advocacy group Sue has sought support from her friends and found strength in her own ability.

Conclusion

I find myself intensely engaged by the work I do, both emotionally and intellectually. At times, it can be very emotionally demanding but it is immensely rewarding and challenging to have the opportunity to become involved and share the highs and lows as people explore their lives and experience health gains and deficits.

Within this chapter I have focused on my work with one individual through two episodes of care. I have identified the many factors that can impinge upon the ability of the individual to overcome incontinence and try to regain continence. Through reflection I have explored my experiences and gained greater insight into the important roles which consistency, collaboration and partnership play when planning and implementing care by utilising a systematic approach. I have identified and explored the complexities within which I work as a nurse in learning disability community nursing. I found reflection on these care episodes challenging and believe I have gained greater insight into my professional practice and its impact upon the person and their family and carers.

References

Atkins, S. & Murphy, K. (1994) Reflective Practice. *Nursing Standard*, **8**(39), 49–54.

Boud, D., Keogh, R. & Walker, D. (1985) *Reflection: turning experience into learning.* Kogan Page, London.

Cameron, C. (1996) Patient compliance: recognition of factors involved and suggestions for promoting compliance within therapeutic regimens. *Journal of Advanced Nursing*, **24**(2), 244–50.

Cardozo, L. (1991) Urinary incontinence in women: have we anything new to offer? *British Medical Journal*, **303**, 1453–57.

Clarke, M. (1991) *Practical Nursing: Hospital and community nursing and health perspectives*. 14th edn. Baillière Tindall, London.

Department of Health (1995) *The Health of The Nation*. HMSO, London.

English National Board for Nursing, Midwifery and Health Visiting (1985) *Caring for people with a mental handicap*. ENB, London.

Getliffe, K. & Dolman, M. (eds) (1997) *Promoting Continence: A clinical and research resource*. Baillière Tindall, London.

Grossman, H.J. (1983) *Classification in mental retardation*. American Association for Mental Deficiency, Washington.

Hussey, L.C. & Gilliland, K. (1989) Compliance, low literacy and locus of control. In: Patient compliance: recognition of factors involved and suggestions for promoting compliance within therapeutic regimens. *Journal of Advanced Nursing*, 24, 244–50.

Johns, C. (1994) Nuances of reflection. *Journal of Clinical Nursing*, 3(2), 71–4.

Kratz, C.R. (ed.) (1979) *The Nursing Process*. Baillière Tindall, London.

Lehne, R.A. (ed.) (1998) *Pharmacology for nursing care*, 3rd edn. W.B. Saunders Company, Philadelphia.

Lewey, J. (1997) Conservative treatment of urinary incontinence. *Nursing Standard*, **12**(8), 45–7.

Lewis, S.J. & Heaton, K.W. (1997) Stool form scale as a useful guide to intestinal transit time. *Scandinavian Journal of Gastroenterology*, Sep; **32**(9), 920–24.

Malone-Lee, J. (1999) Know How: Managing Continence. *Nursing Times*, May, **95**(18), 74–8.

Markwell, S. & Sapsford, R. (1998) Physiotherapy Management of Pelvic Floor Dysfunction. In: Sapsford, R., Bullock-Saxton, J., & Markwell, S. (eds) *Women's Health: A Textbook for Physiotherapists*. W.B. Saunders, London.

Moore, K. & Fader, M. (1999) Promoting continence in the community. *British Journal of Community Nursing*, **4**(1), 36–43.

Norton, C. (1997) Faecal incontinence in adults 2: treatment and management. *British Journal of Nursing*, **6**(1), 23–6.

United Kingdom Central Council for Nursing, Midwifery & Health Visiting (1992) *Code of Professional Conduct*. UKCC, London.

Walsh, M. (1997) (ed) *Watson's clinical nursing and related sciences*, 5th edn. Baillière Tindall, London.

Winney, J. (1998) Constipation. *Nursing Standard*, **13**(11), 49–56.

Withell, B. (2000) A protocol for treating acute constipation in the community setting. *British Journal of Community Nursing*, **5**(3), 114–17.

Chapter 4

Getting the message across: exploring the functions of challenging behaviour

Colin Doyle

A chance encounter

It was a little over 20 years ago that I first came into nursing. I was 19 years old and already had one failed career in the Royal Air Force. I put myself in a strange situation because, back in the early 1980s, the country was in a recession, there were millions of people unemployed and here I was resigning from an electronics course in the belief that I wanted to work with disabled children. This new vision for my future came to me when I was out in a local nightclub. On this particular night some young disabled people and their carers arrived early. They had clearly come out to enjoy themselves before the club got packed. I remember thinking what an extraordinary job the carers seemed to be doing by helping the young people have a good time. The dance floor was full of people, which was unusual so early in the night. I found myself joining in with them with a group of my friends and something inside me said that this was the kind of job for me. Therefore, I set out to find out more.

I was told in the job centre that a local hospital needed staff, so I completed an application form and sent it off. In the mean time I had to return to RAF camp and tell them of my intentions, which did not go down very well. However, on 19 October 1980 I was discharged and the following month I went for an interview to do my nurse training. When I arrived for my interview I had no idea what I was letting myself in for. I wanted to work with children and this was the message I intended to get across during the interview. Although I cannot remember any of the questions I was asked, I remember being shown around afterwards. I realised then, after visiting some of the wards, there were very few children about. Staff were not wearing uniforms, no one was in bed and no one was sick. I knew then that I had blown my interview, I didn't have a clue what the job was about and I was convinced that came across during the interview. As expected, a few days later I received a letter advising me that I had been unsuccessful. However, what did surprise me was that the director of recreation was prepared to offer me a post as a nursing assistant in the residents' social club to give me an opportunity to find out what working with people with learning disabilities was really about. I took the job and three months after starting I was accepted for my training.

I have always remembered that this man gave me an opportunity that was critical to my whole working career. He saw something in me that I was unaware of and gave me a chance. If he hadn't, where would I be now? In those days jobs were hard to come by, let alone a career, and I had been at a major crossroads where the decisions I had taken were life changing. It was his faith in me that made me determined to succeed and to become someone who could make a difference in people's lives.

Culture shock

I remember walking into the grounds on my first day in February 1981 and thinking 'this is great'. Most of the hospital was well hidden from the main road by rows of trees. The atmosphere was tranquil and I thought to myself that in this place you could leave all your outside worries at the gate and could be closeted from the outside world. At the time, the overwhelming sense of self-sufficiency and safety made me feel that it was a terrific place to be. It was somewhat ironic that three years later, as I was coming to the end of my nurse training, I realised that despite all the reasons why I had felt institutional care was good for people with learning disabilities, the opposite was in fact the case. Keeping people enclosed in a self-sufficient community was unacceptable. The paternalism I witnessed was not an acceptable mode of care, and segregation from society did not allow people with learning disabilities to experience the same opportunities that everyone else had.

It was then that I realised that all the reasons why I had liked the place and thought how great it was, had now become the reasons why I hated it. It was an enlightening moment for me because it was then that I realised that I had learned something that would stay with me throughout my career. At the end of 1984, after passing my exams, my first post was as a staff nurse outside the hospital working with children. This fulfilled my vision of helping children to learn and develop. In a small way I also thought that I was helping the closure of the hospital by preventing the children from being admitted. I also remember thinking that I had arrived at where I wanted to be and I thought I knew it all. How wrong I was. My journey had only just started and, 20 years on, that journey is continuing.

Introducing Megan

Megan was the middle child of three, whose family had recently moved into the area. Her parents had no relatives locally and no network of support. Until Megan was 18 months old she had met and achieved all her major development milestones. However, shortly afterwards she became ill and experienced a very high temperature and febrile convulsions. It was following this that her parents noted some marked changes in Megan's behaviour which, unfortunately, paediatricians were unable to diagnose or locate the cause. It was sometime later that she was diagnosed as having Autistic Spectrum Disorder and that this had transpired as a result of this mystery illness.

My involvement with Megan and her family came about following a referral made by the child psychiatrist to the community learning disability team. Whilst this was not an unusual occurrence, the complexities of the situation told me that this would require some careful managing. Megan was only 3 years old when she was referred and, whilst her parents were happy to have a referral made to the community nurses, the fact that the specialist was from a learning disability background was something that appeared less palatable for them. They were pleased to be able to get some practical support and advice but apprehensive about what form that might take. Previous experiences that the family had had from services had not been successful and it was important that my involvement set out to break the chain of dissatisfaction and hostility they felt and expressed.

Megan's behaviour was causing a great deal of distress for the family. She was reported to chew or bite objects and, at times, display pica, which is putting non-food substances such as stones and soil into her mouth. On a number of occasions this had the unfortunate consequence of making her physically ill. Megan was also reported to bite her parents, carers, the children at nursery and siblings and would do so causing significant harm to her victims. These behaviours were beginning to jeopardise Megan's place at the nursery, which was serving as the only acceptable form of respite for her family. This placed further anxiety on both Megan's parents, not only because there was a possibility of Megan being excluded from the nursery but that such a course of action would severely affect her chances of attending mainstream school when the time came.

A complex situation

It had become my job to assess Megan's actions and come up with a strategy to address them. I decided that, whatever I came up with, it had to be something that could be easily understood, implemented and would cause minimum disruption to the family routine. I remember thinking this was not going to be easy and I felt a pressure to succeed. Like most referrals that are received by community learning disability nurses it is only when you begin to conduct your preliminary assessment that it becomes clear that the situation is far more complex than you first thought.

My assessment of the situation began with a comprehensive interview with the parents, where I soon found there was a great deal of unresolved grief being expressed by them both. That is to say, they would talk fondly about how Megan had grown and developed normally through her milestones up until she was 18 months old but when it came to discussing matters beyond the illness the hostility and upset expressed by them both was abundantly clear. They were looking for answers as to why it happened to their child. Why did the services seem so evasive? Why did no one listen to them? Why was there no cure for Megan's condition?

Dealing with parental grief was something I had not been trained to do. This was going to be an unusual situation for me to have to deal with and I was going to have to be as diplomatic as I could to make sure I did not say the wrong thing to the parents and further antagonise the situation. They were grieving for their lost daughter, the one who had been growing and developing so well up until her illness. There was anger towards the health professionals who had failed them in diagnosing and treating Megan's illness, which had now left her disabled. On so many occasions Megan's mother would break down in tears. Sometimes the tears would gently roll down her cheeks and, on other occasions, she would sob almost uncontrollably. At first this made me feel helpless and impotent. There would also be periods of deafening silence where I would hold the mother's hand in comfort or put a gentle arm upon her shoulder as a gesture of support but, on the whole, I still felt humbled by this outpouring of distress and emotion.

Megan's parents refused to accept that she had a learning disability. After all, she had a diagnosis of Autistic Spectrum Disorder and, according to them, Megan was 'trapped' in this disability. In my experience many parents of children with Autistic Spectrum Disorder focus on the fact that not all such individuals have a learning disability and this seems to confuse them. They see that the disability of autism restricts their child's ability to function normally and if somehow they could be reached they would come through it all and begin to lead a normal, independent life. My impression is somewhat supported by the views of experts such as Lorna Wing (1981) and Rita Jordan (2001).

From my encounters with Megan's parents, I felt that I was somehow expected to 'release' Megan from her autism and everything would be all right. Obviously this was impossible but I took their comments and actions as expressions of grief. Nurses cannot afford to ignore expressions of grief like this and I had to give them time and the opportunity to externalise these feelings. At this early stage of involvement the nurse's responses will shape their working relationship with the parents in the months ahead. Given the parents' previous experiences, they wanted to know if I was an ally or a representative of authority.

On my hands and knees

Working with Megan meant that I had to spend time getting to know her and for her to get to know me. I achieved this by spending time with her at her home where we would spend two or three hours playing around on the floor with her toys. She was particularly interested in books and enjoyed listening to nursery rhymes, so that was much of what we did. I needed to carry out some assessment work if I was going to determine some hypothesis to work with. For some people, assessment can conjure up an image of endless form-filling but that is not always the case. Nurses use observation of what happens but also what doesn't happen.

One aspect of her behaviour I focused on was how Megan communicated her needs. It was clear that she had no verbal communication, so how did she achieve this? I observed that she used her mother as a natural extension of herself. If she wanted a drink, she would take her by the hand and lead her to the kitchen or, if a drink was close by, Megan would give her a cup. When the music tape stopped she led her mother to the machine to get her to turn it over or put on a new one. Whilst this should not be interpreted as maladaptive behaviour in any way, the frequency of such a demand upon her mother was such that it would place pressure upon her to understand what Megan wanted and, therefore, would need addressing. At this early stage I thought that one of the strategies that would ultimately reduce the need for Megan to place this demand upon her mother would be to develop and improve her verbal communication ability.

Megan would show no interest in her brother or sister as they played around her. Even when they took books or toys from her she would just get another one. The only time Megan reacted to them was when they made demands on their mother and Megan also wanted her attention. These were the times that I observed her climbing. Megan would literally climb all over her mother, the furniture and along the bannisters to the stairs. She would get herself into so many awkward positions it was inevitable that from time to time she would fall. When the family went out, Megan would want to be carried or travel in a pushchair. She was too big for the pushchair and too heavy to carry for long periods, and as a result would just sit down on the floor. Outdoors, Megan would persistently attempt to pick up things from the floor and put them in her mouth. Indoors, she would pick crumbs from the floor and anything else that had been discarded by the family.

I noted that Megan's biting, although not malicious, appeared to have significant communicative power. I hypothesised that this behaviour was being maintained by its use as an effective tool to communicate her need to 'get away' or for someone to leave her alone. This strategy worked, especially with other children. For someone with no speech, Megan had developed some effective techniques for herself that had the desired effect and, the more they worked, the more reinforcing they became.

The pica behaviour is another example. I believed that Megan had no desire to eat non-edible objects but, every now and again, she would be successful in picking something up that was edible. Donnellan *et al.* (1988) pointed out that intermittent reinforcement is the strongest type of reinforcement of behaviour. Megan's pica behaviour was following an intermittent reinforcement pattern. This was quite different from the mouthing behaviour of putting toys into her mouth. This appeared to be more 'self-stimulatory': that is, it was her way of playing. My observations also indicated that this was more likely to occur if Megan was alone.

Much of this information was gathered during my visits to the family home but it was also important for Megan's parents to become involved in the assessment process to help them feel included and, it was hoped, to help them develop new insights into their daughter's actions. I sat down with them and explained that I wanted them to record Megan's actions over a period of two hours when it was more likely that she would engage in some of the behaviours we were interested in. I also asked her parents to note what was happening before and after the behaviour in question. The key here was to work out the function of the behaviour. Everything we do has a reason or function and Megan was doing what she was doing for a reason. Therefore, we would need to piece together the recording charts and come up with some suggestions for the function of Megan's behaviour. We also needed information that would let us know if Megan's health would be affected by any of her actions. For example, some of the non-foodstuffs could potentially be very dangerous.

Establishing priorities

Following many hours of observation and making sense of the information, the time came to prioritise actions that would help Megan. Where there are different expectations between those involved, this process needs negotiating. In Megan's case everyone was in agreement that there was a need to ensure that Megan's physical health was maintained and that all efforts were made to ensure she did not suffer from any avoidable illnesses and accidents. We also felt that some efforts needed to be made to prevent any further deterioration in her relationship with her sister because we believed that a positive rapport between them would help them both, as well as alleviate the distress this was having upon the family as a unit. We translated these decisions into a set of aims which were:

- To reduce the frequency of Megan mouthing toys and objects that she might pick up or handle.
- To reduce the frequency of Megan eating non-food substances (pica).
- To redirect Megan's skill in climbing, into an activity and environment that was more appropriate.
- To improve Megan's relationship with her sister so that their time together was positive and mutually rewarding.

These goals were written down and detailed in an intervention plan. The key phrases here were 'to reduce the frequency of' because there is always a need to aim for something that was achievable. We were also going to 're-direct', instead of eliminate. This is because we have to accept that, in Megan's case, she likes to climb and if it is something she likes to do then trying to stop it all together would be almost impossible. Instead, what we chose to do was to give it value and also value Megan's choice by giving it validity and trying to teach her what she can safely and appropriately climb. The principle behind such an approach is embraced in positive programming principles and is to be found in work by Donnellan *et al.* (1988).

What was not forgotten was the fact that Megan's relationship with her older sister was deteriorating and that needed to be repaired and improved. Megan's sister was feeling that everything centred on Megan and that the family could not do the things other families did because of Megan's disability. She felt she could not bring her friends home after school because of Megan and that she did not get invited to other children's homes because of her sister and she could not always have the time and attention from her mother because of her need to see to Megan. We set about this by helping her sister to understand some of Megan's needs and the reasons why she behaved as she did. We would also try to encourage both parents to set aside quality time for all their children and make sure that when deviations occurred to this routine they were understood and appreciated by the other children and that they were kept to a minimum. This was going to be a difficult task, especially given that Megan's sister was only six years old herself and that her parents had already established a strong routine around Megan and had until this point thought it had been working well.

Taking each target skill in turn, there was a need to outline the protocol or procedure to be followed. This required a step-by-step description of what needed to be done, and how it would be implemented. Fundamental to this process was the devising of a recording system because, as time progressed, achievements, no matter how small, needed to be identified and recognised. This was going to provide the measure of change and become the baseline material that each week's progress would be measured against. For each of our identified goals a detailed intervention and strategy was designed for implementation.

Putting priorities into action

Before describing a strategy that would reduce the frequency of the target behaviours, it was important to be sure of the current frequency. This would help to determine the level at which the behaviour was occurring and set out some of the conditions in which they were more likely to occur. The results of observations for three target behaviours are shown in Figure 4.1.

These results were obtained over a 60-minute time period of observation. For each of the recorded behaviours, there was a significant reduction in the frequency of occurrence when I engaged Megan in an activity.

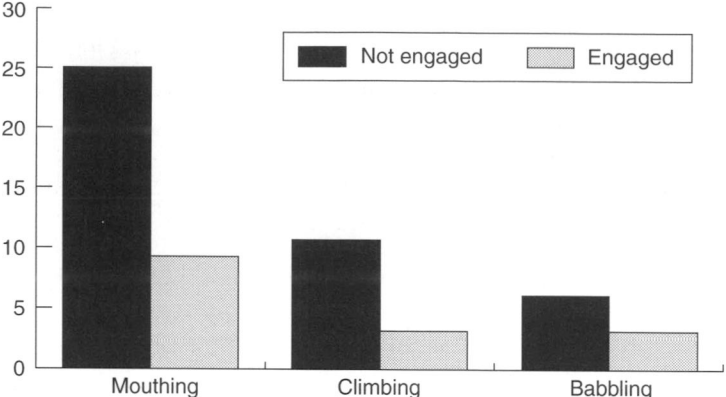

Figure 4.1   Frequency of three behaviours.

The results in Figure 4.2 were also obtained over a 60-minute observation period. For each of the recorded activities, there was a significant reduction in the frequency of 'neutral' activity and a corresponding increase in alternative participatory activities when I engaged Megan in an activity. These pre-liminary findings appeared to indicate that when Megan had her time structured and supported by others, she was less likely to engage in the target behaviour and more likely to play constructively with meaningful outcomes. From this data, there was a need to approach this behaviour from two pro-cedures that included a reactive strategy and a proactive strategy (Donnellan *et al.*, 1988).

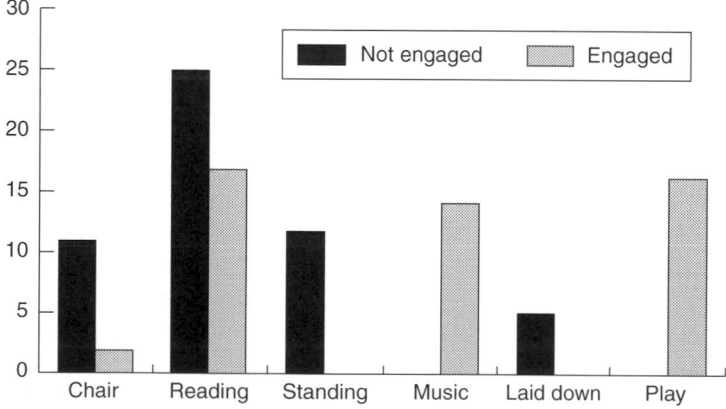

Figure 4.2   Frequency of behaviours, shown in Figure 4.1, when engaged in an activity vs. unengaged.

Reactive strategy

This was a strategy that was designed to stop the target behaviour from continuing immediately. It would prevent Megan from maintaining that behaviour, but it would not prevent her from doing so again at a later point in time. This was to be a short-term strategy that was intended to have short-term benefits. It would, of course, reduce the possibility of Megan becoming ill from eating non-food substances, but its purpose was not to address the problem in its entirety.

In this instance, Megan was to be told 'No', in a strong and firm manner. This would stop her from continuing to put an item in her mouth, but she might of course switch to an alternative item. It was decided that it would appropriate at the outset to allow Megan to 'mouth' one toy or item. This would allow her to continue the behaviour if she felt the desire to do so but in the long term it would be gradually shaped away from what she was doing. Once this item was selected it did not change and neither was she permitted to mouth anything else. The availability of other potential mouthing objects also needed to be restricted because their mere presence could have acted as an antecedent for this behaviour to occur. Whilst there may appear to be problems with consistency of approach, the belief that we were addressing the target behaviour and in fact shaping the behaviour to be more manageable ensured that the approach was adhered to. Megan would gradually associate the mouthing of a particular toy to be safe and that a different response followed when she repeated this with other toys.

We were conscious of the need to avoid placing too much emphasis upon negative interaction for inappropriate mouthing. We wanted to reward and reinforce Megan when she engaged with an item appropriately. She needed to be praised and told for example, 'well done Megan, that's right, this is how that works'. On the occasions when Megan did not know how to 'play' with a particular toy, we needed to show her what to do. In addition, this approach would be used following each occurrence that she had to be told 'No', because she had mouthed something.

Proactive strategy

This strategy was going to be more long term in its implementation and in its benefits to Megan. I suggested that Megan's behaviour could be altered by reducing the opportunity for the behaviour to occur and to structure her activities so that she did not engage in self-stimulatory activities quite so often. This would be very demanding upon whoever carried this out. However, Megan engaged in activities where she demonstrated that she would sit and listen and watch the TV or listen to her music centre. Megan was periodically given the time and space to do this because she had already demonstrated through assessment that she was less likely to mouth objects to a high degree if there was background music playing that she liked.

Megan's day was to be structured into activities in order to reduce the opportunity that she had to mouth objects. Briefly, this included:

- Periodic removal of the stimulating items that were likely to increase the frequency of the behaviour occurring. These would be toys that she frequently mouthed that were small enough to put into her mouth.

- The toys would only be available when a structured activity that reinforced their appropriate use was enacted. As was previously stated, one item would be left for her to use in this way, especially if she was likely to become distressed. The aim was to not only reduce the frequency of mouthing, but also to produce a reduction of the type of objects that she would be likely to mouth.

- We planned to make use of musical toys that would play a tune or music when keys were pressed. Megan appeared to enjoy very much the farm animal noises on a toy that we played with and this would be one toy we would use regularly. A small keyboard, drum or tambourine was also an idea we had to introduce, where Megan would make her own music.

- Naturally, the use of her music audiotapes was something we set out to utilise, particularly during self-structured activities. A natural extension to this was for her to watch musical videos, such as those with nursery rhymes and those of her favourite characters that were depicted in some of her books.

- Another source of self-structured play would come from her books. This is something that Megan initiated, but would also be used as an activity that she could be persuaded to gradually allow others to join in with. This was something we had hoped that the whole family could participate in and be the start of re-establishing a harmonious relationship with her sister. At nursery she had been using 'body awareness' audiotapes which she had indicated that she enjoyed through her body language and facial expression.

- A whole collection of noises, especially voices, would be made into a recording for her to listen to on tape. Noises had their fascination for Megan and this was yet another way that we could exploit her strength. We had managed to find this out during our observations at home and from feedback from the nursery staff.

- Because of Megan's natural desire to climb, some kind of appropriate climbing frame or opportunity was proposed. This would mean that any activity that took place of this nature needed to be well supervised. The local children's recreational soft play area that provided soft play equipment was also a resource that we would take up. It was anticipated that such an activity would need to be structured because of Megan's difficulty in self-directed play but again it was something the whole family could participate in together. It also had the added benefit that this is a gross motor activity and therefore Megan would be less likely to come across materials that could require her to use her fine motor skills in the same way as picking up items and putting them in her mouth.

- For set periods of the day, small bowls of appropriate food items would be strategically placed about the playroom. This would allow Megan the opportunity to snack if she felt the need to do so, and the opportunity to reward and reinforce appropriate behaviour would present itself at the same time.

Whenever any food fell to the floor, such as crisps that got dropped or biscuits that got broken, I strongly advised that they were cleared up by vacuuming without delay. This would reduce the opportunity for Megan to find such items lying around, and then break the intermittent reinforcement that she experienced whenever she picked up food from the floor. On a practical level, something like a portable vacuum cleaner was found more convenient to do this.

The cornerstone to success was going to be the reward and reinforcement of appropriate behaviours and the 'over learning' that would take place whenever the target behaviour presented. The message here needed to be strong and consistent. In order to gain a measure of the progress that was achieved, I arranged that a one-hour period of observation and recording took place every two weeks, over a six-week period and was then reviewed. The recordings would provide me with a snapshot measure of the progress and achievement.

In addition, Megan liked and enjoyed physical contact with other people, for example playing games such as tickling and rough and tumble. Megan would react well to this type of activity by frequently exploding into bouts of laughter, indicating great pleasure and excitement. Megan particularly enjoyed going swimming and she would spend time playing in the shower and the bath whenever the opportunity presented itself. She also appeared to receive a great deal of pleasure from visual stimulation. She would spend time watching the trees and clouds moving. She particularly enjoyed the sensation of the wind on her face. Because Megan had shown that animals gave her a certain amount of pleasure, particularly when she had been on visits to farms and zoos, it was decided to try and explore the possibility of her going for horse riding lessons.

Outcomes

It is always good practice for nurses to evaluate their work at regular intervals. This is especially true when nurses are working on long-term matters and when progress may be slow. It is surprising when you look back over what has actually happened and see the measures of progress that have been made. This makes both the family feel enthusiastic but can also revitalise the nurse. In turn, this helps to maintain motivation and see a more positive future. As a result of the interventions that I put in place and that the family carried out we were able to identify the following achievements with Megan:

- Megan was less likely to engage in inappropriate chewing of objects whenever her time was structured. The availability of potential mouthing objects also affected the frequency of mouthing and she was less likely to engage in this behaviour when objects were unavailable.

- Megan was less likely to lick toys or objects during structured activity, but was more likely to present with this behaviour when she was looking at books.

- It was found that Megan was likely to put her fingers into her mouth when engaged in structured activities and this may have been because during structured sessions she was unable to easily seek out an object to mouth, so instead mouthed her fingers.

- Megan had shown that she was less likely to engage in hand waving behaviours when she was occupied, something that was not always received with pleasure by her parents. This behaviour had increased in frequency and duration throughout the intervention period.

- Megan did not climb very much at all at nursery and generally did not do so when she was otherwise engaged at home. It was more likely to occur when Megan was left in an unstructured environment and from our observations appeared to occur more often at home.

- One of the pleasing outcomes had been the obvious increase in Megan initiating contact with other people. This had increased dramatically. Megan would also engage a person with eye contact more frequently and she appeared more observant of the things around her and more balanced in her posture.

- Megan was vocalising more frequently, and would do so more often in unstructured activities. This may have been because during structured activities Megan saw herself as fulfilling and playing a role led by others. However, during unstructured activity she would be free to express herself in other ways. Megan was also showing signs that she was able to respond appropriately to verbal instructions.

- Megan appeared to be demonstrating an improved ability to explore and decide what things can do around her. She appeared to occupy herself through play more appropriately and did not always discard toys she came across, many times choosing to explore them appropriately. An interesting development was when Megan decided to stand up a toy dwarf she had at home when it had fallen over or whenever she saw it laid on its side: a point where she recognised the appropriate nature of this toy.

- Megan was also observed to be smiling more frequently. As she smiled she would sometimes glance over towards someone and laugh, resulting in her facial expression becoming more animated and expressive.

Conclusions

Megan was now able to discriminate between objects, choosing particular ones that she preferred to put into her mouth. Initially, the availability of such objects was high, as was the presence of foodstuffs that functioned as an intermittent reinforcer that had made their way to the floor. When they were available, the effect on the pica behaviour was to increase their frequency, therefore rewarding and reinforcing it. When they were unavailable, the effect was to reduce its occurrence because no effective reward was available for Megan.

Megan's cooperation and her interaction with others improved. Megan's parents and I concluded that she had become more assertive about her own needs. Megan still very much enjoyed her books, music and videos. When engaged in these activities, she was less likely to mouth toys or objects. Megan became more likely to make sounds when engaged in unstructured activities but at the same time more likely to mouth toys. Diversion techniques that prevented the mouthing behaviour from occurring or engaging Megan in an alternative way that was inconsistent with the target behaviour had an encouraging effect in reducing the likelihood of mouthing occurring.

The indicators had been that Megan benefited from a structured educational play timetable and responded well to direction. When she received one-to-one support she was less likely to put herself at risk by putting objects into her mouth and, as such, these behaviours became self-managing. I recognised that there existed a continued need to be aware that the previous problems regarding 'mouthing' were always likely to re-establish themselves. It was one thing to change the current management procedure to acknowledge the conditions that were likely to increase the possibility of this behaviour re-occurring, but rigorously controlling those conditions was another.

I went on to work on a number of other areas with Megan, that included continence skills, but the work we did together during those first months would always have an influence upon me. It was a steep learning curve for me as I came to realise the complexities of the challenges Megan presented, but together we came out the other side. Megan's relationship with her sister showed little signs of improvement despite our efforts. Maybe that was something to do with her age and the possibility that some resentment may have built up towards Megan by her because of the time demands she made on their mother.

Fond memories

As a learning disability nurse, there is a need to reflect on your work and try to put your practice experiences into context from time to time. This can allow nurses to see connections between aspects of their role and enables them to refresh their practice. I have found that learning disability nurses have to think laterally and see how the complexities of situations all fit together and what strategies can help people. Megan was a joy to work with and I appreciated playing some part in her life. The achievements detailed here are her achievements, ones in which I had the opportunity to share with her and her parents. Whilst I came in to the home and advised and did some hands-on work, it was inevitably her immediate family who meticulously carried out the intervention. It should be remembered that the work of a learning disability nurse requires them to work together with the individual, the family and others because they are unlikely to succeed if they work alone. The individual's and the family's motivation can be very strong because they inevitably want the best for their son or daughter. I am glad I realised that in Megan's case and harnessed this motivation and turned it into goodwill.

References

Donnellan, A., LaVigna, G.W., Negri-Shoultz, N. & Fassbender, L.L. (1988) *Progress without Punishment. Effective Approaches for Learners with Behaviour Problems.* Teachers College Press, Columbia University, New York.

Jordan, R. (2001). *Autism with Severe Learning Difficulties.* Souvenir Press Ltd, The Guernsey Press Co Ltd, Human Horizon Series, London.

Wing, L. (1981) *Autistic Children. A Guide for Parents.* Redwood Burn Ltd, London.

Further reading

Pace, G.M. & Toyer, E.A. (2000) The effects of a vitamin supplement on the pica of a child with severe mental retardation. *Journal of Applied Behavioural Analysis.* **33**(4), 619–22.

Wallace, J. & Alvarez, O. (1999) Pica and iron deficiency. A case report. *Wisconsin Medical Journal,* **98**(3), 54–6.

Wolfensberger, W. (1983) Social Role Valourization: A Proposed New Term for the Principle of Normalization. *Mental Retardation,* **21**(6), 234–9.

Chapter 5

The purpose and practice of learning disability nursing

Gwen Moulster and John Turnbull

Introduction

It is safe to assume that the most frequently asked question in relation to learning disability nursing is 'what do learning disability nurses do?' The question is honest and straightforward enough, yet its answer is inevitably more complex. Despite their separate aims and content, many of the chapters in this book already provide answers to this question. However, this chapter is dedicated to providing an overview of the purpose and practice of learning disability nursing and critically reflecting on practice by asking:

- What are the aims of learning disability nursing?
- How do learning disability nurses achieve their aims?

The chapter will draw upon three sources of information to answer these questions. First, the chapter will explore some of the key statements made about learning disability nursing from authorities such as the Department of Health, Royal College of Nursing and bodies responsible for nurse education. Second, there have been a modest number of research projects into learning disability nursing. Although this chapter cannot provide a comprehensive literature review, it will draw out common themes in relation to the purpose and practice of nursing. Third, some of the accounts of practice in this book will be used to supplement and illustrate key points about practice.

The purpose of learning disability nursing

The origins of modern definitions

This section will consider what it is that learning disability nurses set out to achieve. Despite the persistent questions about the aims of learning disability nursing, the literature reveals no shortage of descriptions. Inevitably, these descriptions have varied over the years to accommodate professional and policy imperatives, as well as perceptions of the needs of people with learning disabilities and their families. However, contemporary definitions of practice can be traced to the 1980s. The 1982 syllabus for learning disability nurse education (English National Board, 1982) put forward a bold statement about learning disability nursing by incorporating a philosophy of care and support for people with learning disabilities that would be recognisable to today's professionals in the field. The preface to the syllabus recognised that people with learning disabilities have the same human value as anyone else in society and that they have a right and a need to live like other people in the community. The syllabus went on to state that the role of learning disability nurses was to use their unique professional skills to support them to achieve this.

The Chief Nursing Officer reinforced this view in her declaration on the role of the learning disability nurse in 1985 (Department of Health and Social Security, 1985). The nurse's role was described as being one of providing individualised care to people with learning disabilities and their families and collaborating with others to create alternatives to hospital care. The definition stopped short of using phrases such as 'a normal life' or 'ordinary living', though the Chief Nursing Officer referred readers to the 1982 syllabus and its philosophy for further information. Three months prior to this declaration the English National Board (1985) issued a circular on the role and function of the learning disability nurse. This circular asserted that all people with learning disabilities should have access to the skills of a learning disability nurse. The circular also went into some detail about the skills nurses were expected to display that included teaching, training and communicating with people with learning disabilities. The circular also claimed that nurses should be available to provide advice and support to parents and other paid carers.

The themes of independence and equality of opportunity within these statements were encapsulated in a more concise definition of learning disability nursing developed for the Project 2000 framework for nurse education introduced in 1987 (United Kingdom Central Council, 1987). This definition stated that:

> 'The function of the nurse for people with mental handicap is to directly and skilfully assist the individual and his/her family, whatever the handicap, in the acquisition, development and maintenance of those skills that, given the necessary ability, would be performed unaided and to do this in such a way as to enable independence to be gained as rapidly and as fully as possible in an environment that maintains a quality of life that would be acceptable to fellow citizens of the same age.'

This definition is actually an adaptation of Virginia Henderson's definition of nursing that she developed in 1961 (Henderson, 1961), but fits in with the theme of maximising the independence of the individual.

Other descriptions of the role of the learning disability nurse at this time, particularly from the Royal College of Nursing (1989, 1992), simply reinforced the messages from official sources such as the English National Board and the Chief Nursing Officer. These definitions were supported by what little research about learning disability nursing existed during the 1980s. Valerie Hall and Oliver Russell, from the University of Bristol, had been commissioned by the Department of Health to investigate the emerging role of the community learning disability nurse and the reports of their findings are summarised in Hall and Russell (1985a,b). In these studies, nurses describe their role as supporting people to lead independent and normal lives in the community. The researchers' observations of nurses confirmed this view and also supported the subsequent descriptions of nurses' skills as consisting of advising and counselling individuals and family members as well as developing training programmes for people with learning disabilities to increase their everyday living skills.

An endorsement of the nurse's role as a leader was provided by Leonard's (1988) research into the quality of care of children with learning disabilities. Leonard reports that:

> 'The most shining examples of inspiring home leadership and dynamic management were all people originally nurse-trained in long stay mental handicap hospitals.'

This leadership and management role of the learning disability nurse is one that used to be underplayed by official descriptions of learning disability nursing in the 1980s, which tended to concentrate on clinical, or 'hands-on' skills and abilities. Given the dispersed nature of services in the community and the steady growth of small residential facilities throughout the 1980s and 1990s, many nurses found themselves managing and leading small teams of staff in these services. Therefore, many learning disability nurses had to acquire and demonstrate their leadership skills at a much earlier stage in their career compared to their counterparts from other branches of nursing. It is possible that nursing curricula were geared much more towards the needs of acute nurses who would not need to take responsibility as soon as their learning disability colleagues. If this is accurate, it adds value to the personal characteristics of learning disability nurses and, possibly, their capacity to reflect on and learn from practice. More recently, documents such as *Continuing the Commitment* (Kay *et al.*, 1995), and research studies such as Alaszewski *et al.* (2001), have called for a strengthening of the management component of nurse education.

A change of direction

Definitions and descriptions of the purpose of learning disability nursing took on a different complexion in the early 1990s. The NHS and Community Care

Act (Department of Health, 1990) was almost certainly responsible for this change, for two reasons. First, the Act called for a sharp distinction between health and social care responsibilities within services. Second, the introduction of the internal market for healthcare prompted many professions and services to describe themselves in more marketable terms. The All Wales Nursing Group for People with a Mental Handicap provided an early indication of a change in thinking about how to describe learning disability nursing (All Wales Nursing Group, 1992). This document put learning disability nursing firmly within the context of healthcare. By using the World Health Organization's holistic definition of health, rather than a biophysiological one, the group stated that the purpose of learning disability nursing was working towards health gain for individuals with learning disabilities. In addition, the group included in their definition more familiar objectives such as encouraging more normal patterns of living and maximising individual potential.

If the members of the All Wales Nursing Group had one eye on the emerging marketplace for healthcare when writing their document, the gaze of the Royal College of Nursing seems to have been firmly focused on it during the early 1990s. In 1994, the Royal College of Nursing published a guide to learning disability nursing for purchasers (Royal College of Nursing, 1994). Like the All Wales Nursing Group, this description committed learning disability nurses to work to improve health gain for service users and informed purchasers of care that nurses achieved this because they could:

- Carry out assessment and diagnoses.
- Plan developmental care regimes.
- Prevent ill health and promote health.
- Provide rehabilitation and remedial therapy.
- Provide physical care.

Although many nurses might have agreed with this list, the distinctive aspect of the document is that the value base of nursing is referred to only at the end of the document where nurses are described as also having a role to play in advocating for people with learning disabilities.

The theme of health gain featured prominently in *Continuing the Commitment* (Kay *et al.*, 1995) and its accompanying document for health and social care commissioners entitled *Meeting Needs through Targeting Skills* (Department of Health, 1995). These descriptions of learning disability nursing were the eagerly awaited outcome of a project commissioned by the Chief Nursing Officer into the role of the learning disability nurse. The documents put forward a clear value base for working with people with learning disabilities that was to work with individuals to strengthen their autonomy and develop more valued lifestyles. During the course of the project, 200 examples of best practice in learning disability nursing had been submitted to the project leaders, from which the following definition of purpose was developed (Department of Health, 1995, p. 7):

'The purpose of nursing for people with learning disability is to work in partnership with the individual to improve his or her personal autonomy. This is achieved by seeking to:

- Mitigate the effects of disability.
- Achieve optimum health.
- Facilitate access to and encourage involvement in local communities.
- Increase personal competence.
- Maximise choice.
- Enhance the contribution of others either formally or informally involved in supporting the individual.'

This definition and the description in *Continuing the Commitment* attracted the broad approval of the profession, not least because it emphasised the healthcare role of the nurse (Birchenall, 1996). It also addressed what had become an area of controversy over the use of the word 'independence' to describe the aim of learning disability nursing. As Jeanette Thompson and Sharon Pickering discuss in Chapter 9, society places such great value on the concept of independence that to be thought of as dependent on anyone is to be considered weak or not resourceful. The fact of the matter is that people cannot live without each other and a more accurate and appropriate phrase to use is *inter*-dependence. It was also thought to be more accurate to believe that what people with learning disabilities said they needed was greater choice and control, hence the substitution of the word independence with autonomy when describing the aims of learning disability nursing.

Continuing the Commitment probably remains the most comprehensive description by Government of learning disability nursing. However, whether or not this document, and others produced during the 1990s, are the most accurate representation of learning disability nursing is still open to question. A major issue is whether the healthcare role of the learning disability nurse was something that began to appear in documents because of political expediency or whether nurses had been playing and could continue to play a key role in improving the health of people with learning disabilities.

Research into learning disability nursing since 1990 provides a mixed view. One of the major conclusions from an extensive study by Clifton *et al.* (1992), was that learning disability nursing practice reflected current philosophies of supporting people with learning disabilities. According to the researchers, this meant that nurses were supporting the rights and choices of individuals and supporting them to live in community settings. It is interesting that managers and professional colleagues of nurses who were interviewed as part of this research highlighted nurses' competence at dealing with health related issues, though this aspect of practice was not highlighted by nurses themselves at interview. In another large study by Norman *et al.* (1996) expert informants were asked to report on the relevance of nurse education in learning disability. Part of the study included exploring the current purpose of learning disability nursing with them. It is interesting that most respondents identified promoting autonomy, supporting self-advocacy and assessing need as the main functions of the nurse but hardly any of them mentioned health related functions.

Owen Barr's survey (1994) of community teams in Northern Ireland adds to the picture in that the 35 community nurses who responded reported that their main reasons for referral included problems related to epilepsy, physical impairment or mental health. Barr's findings were later supported by a small-scale study by Stewart and Todd (2001) into the purpose and function of learning disability nursing in which nurses claimed to have knowledge and skills in health promotion, knowledge of drugs, knowledge of research, managing continence, hygiene, epilepsy, problem solving and crisis management. In the same year Blackmore (2001) reported on a project that explored eight learning disability nurses' experiences of advocacy. Although it was not the aim of this research to explore the purpose of learning disability nursing, respondents saw their role as one of supporting individuals to make decisions, to create supportive communication environments for advocacy to happen and to help individuals access advocates.

Bradley (1999) carried out an interesting piece of research in which he gave small numbers of social workers, community nurses and informal carers information on hypothetical individuals with learning disabilities and asked them to identify their needs. Despite the artificial nature of this approach, Bradley discovered that, whereas nurses were good at identifying a greater breadth of need than the other two groups, they failed to identify opportunities for health promotion. A study focused on 32 individuals with learning disabilities and their encounters with learning disability nurses by Hunt *et al.* (2001) yielded some interesting findings. In this study nurses took part in identifying unmet health needs and provided advice on medication and other health related issues.

Similarly, in a survey of community nurse managers in 170 NHS Trusts (Mobbs *et al.*, 2002), managers reported that 'health monitoring' was amongst the most frequent activity engaged in by learning disability nurses with 'health promotion' the sixth most frequent, followed by 'health screening' in eighth place. Of course, it must be remembered that this information relies upon managers' impressions of nursing activity rather than actual practice, but it suggests that nurses are often engaged in health related activity. Curiously, and in contrast to long-lasting statements about the purpose of learning disability nursing, this survey had little to report on activity that might be described as promoting choice or control by people with learning disabilities.

A large-scale study by Alaszewski *et al.* (2001) had the opportunity to explore the authenticity of statements regarding the health related role of the learning disability nurse. The study set out to explore the educational preparation of learning disability nurses, part of which included exploring current nursing practice. When asked, nurses reported that management, liaising with others and education were the most important components of their work. This was largely confirmed by direct observation by the researchers who developed four main categories of nursing activity arising from their study. Under the category of 'user and carer support', for two-thirds of the time, nurses were observed to be involved in health surveillance. Once again, when service users and carers were asked about the value of learning disability nursing, they reported that the clinical aspects of the nurses' role, such as blood pressure monitoring or giving of medication, were a distinctive feature of their practice.

Summary

To briefly summarise this section, the research literature and key documents suggest that a fundamental purpose of learning disability nursing is to promote the autonomy of people with learning disabilities. A more recently articulated goal has been the promotion of the health of people with learning disabilities. However, some of the literature suggests that nurses themselves may not regard this as an aspect of their practice, or that nurses are not familiar with describing their actions in terms of healthcare. This raises complex political issues about the role of the learning disability nurse. First, it could be argued that their healthcare role has been emphasised in order to keep them within the family of nursing. Second, it could have been emphasised because of the considerable unmet healthcare needs of people with learning disabilities (Kerr *et al.*, 1996).

Whatever people's views are about these issues, the research seems to suggest that nurses have the potential to fulfil a specialist healthcare purpose. A key issue for learning disability nurses would be to ensure that this role enhances their capacity to support the rights and independence of people with learning disabilities. Added to this is the need to ensure that nurses are equipped with the necessary skills to fulfil this function (Alaszewski *et al.*, 2001). Finally, nurses could link their multiple roles by developing and utilising frameworks and models for their practice. One such model, developed by John Aldridge, is included in the penultimate chapter of this book.

Understanding nursing practice

A breadth of knowledge

Moving on from this discussion about the aims of learning disability nursing, this section will explore how nurses go about achieving those and also discuss whether it is possible to describe how effective they are at this. Several reports have referred to the breadth of knowledge within learning disability nursing as a key factor in their success in working with people with learning disabilities. The Cullen Report (Four Chief Nursing Officers, 1991) into learning disability nursing not only drew attention to the breadth but also the depth of nursing skills that enabled some nurses to specialise in supporting people with challenging behaviour and people with multiple disabilities. This was confirmed by the extensive observations of nurses carried out by Clifton *et al.* (1992), as part of their research. Also, in their interviews with managers in the health service as well as the independent sector, both sets of respondents reported that they valued the comprehensive knowledge of learning disability nurses that enabled them to carry out a range of functions. Likewise, families of service users in the study by Alaszewski *et al.* (2001) praised nurses' knowledge of learning disability and associated conditions such as epilepsy, continence and physical impairment. In this study, nurses themselves also recognised that they had the knowledge to fulfil a number of roles ranging from health promotion to managing staff.

This breadth of knowledge could be a reason why nurses and their colleagues report that they are accomplished at carrying out assessment of need. As pointed out in the previous section, Bradley (1999) concluded that nurses were more effective than social workers and lay people at identifying a breadth of health and social care need. The Royal College of Nursing took up this point by proposing that nurses would be ideally placed to become care managers (Royal College of Nursing, 1992). This Royal College of Nursing document, as well as *Continuing the Commitment* (Kay *et al.*, 1995), identified assessment as a key function of the learning disability nurse and extended this to other executive functions of care such as evaluation and service quality monitoring. The breadth of nurses' knowledge could also serve the purpose of providing a sound platform on which to build more specialist practice. The Royal College of Nursing put forward this argument, amongst others, in response to the recommendation of the Consensus Conference Panel that learning disability nursing should no longer be a separate branch of nursing (cited in Brown, 1994). This argument has never been tested but it is a popular one amongst those who want to maintain the branch programme in learning disability.

On the other hand, there are others who see the breadth of knowledge and skills in learning disability nursing as a weakness. The argument put forward here is that it creates a practitioner who is a 'Jack (or Jill) of all trades but master (or mistress) of none'. Given that the research is broadly complimentary about the nurse's role, this feeling may have more to do with more general feelings of nurses about how they are valued than a comment on their effectiveness. It is also worth pointing out that this versatility and breadth of practice seem to be qualities possessed by the profession rather than the individual professional. In other words, the education and preparation of learning disability nurses contains the ingredients to produce a variety of different practitioners.

A unique role?

A key issue that has often been raised in relation to nurses' knowledge is how distinctive it is in relation to their professional colleagues and unqualified support staff. In the study undertaken by Alaszewski *et al.* (2001), unqualified support workers questioned the uniqueness of learning disability nurses' knowledge and skills. Having a unique body of knowledge and skills is traditionally seen as the hallmark of professional practice (Moline, 1986). Unfortunately, the little research into the area of learning disability nursing practice suggests that learning disability nurses do not have a body of knowledge or skills that is unique.

Clifton *et al.* (1992) were commissioned to investigate the transferability of learning disability nurses' skills from hospital to community and the distinctiveness of those skills. They concluded that there were no skills that were the exclusive preserve of nurses. However, after reaching this conclusion, the researchers went on to assert that it was the combination of knowledge and skills of the learning disability nurse that was distinctive. The researchers saw this combination as nurses' added value and labelled this phenomenon as the 'skills plus' factor. A similar view was expressed by Raynes *et al.* (1994) who noted a 'quality effect' of employing learning disability nurses as managers of residential facilities. In his investigation into learning disability nursing, Cullen (Four Chief Nursing Officers, 1991) also expressed an opinion on the issue of nurses' unique body of knowledge by commenting that no profession could lay claim to a skill that could not be performed by someone else. Moline (1986) points out that a unique body of knowledge is not the sole determinant of professional status. If this were so, then plumbers and electricians would lay claim to the title. Therefore, perhaps learning disability nurses should not get unduly anxious about this aspect of their practice.

The art and science of practice

Moving on from this, it may be that professional practice has more to do with the level of knowledge and reasoning applied to a given situation than its distinctiveness. This has created a problem for learning disability nurses. For example, Cullen (1991) remarked that he believed that learning disability nurses displayed some 'low level' skills, though he did not go on to describe what they were. Turnbull (1995) later referred to a growing assumption amongst some that supporting individuals with learning disabilities required few high level skills or specialist knowledge.

Schon (1987) has pointed out the dangers of making judgements about professional action based on limited information. He put forward the view that many apparently small or insignificant actions could actually be the outcome of complex thinking, problem solving and decision-making, and could also be very important to an individual client or patient. For instance, Peter Dawson's silences (see Chapter 6) and the things that he decided *not* to say are probably more important than what he actually said to Judith and it may have been this that encouraged her to speak out more. Rebecca Welsh (see Chapter 12) made some subtle and deliberate changes to her posture in order to encourage Tristan's mother to express her feelings, perhaps because Rebecca recognised that this was a crucial point in her relationship with the family. As Schon pointed out, these examples illustrate the need to explore the context in which practice takes place in order to generate a three dimensional picture of practice.

Schon believed that these small and subtle aspects of professional practice are indications of the artistry of individual nurses and other practitioners. According to Schon, however, the artistry of practice has been overshadowed by the dominance of technical and scientific knowledge in our society. The technical and scientific view of the world believes that all reality is capable of being measured, explained and ordered into a set of laws which then leads to a society which can be better controlled (Marks-Maran, 1999). This type of thinking has been responsible for many advances in society and, in the field of healthcare, it has provided solutions to many of the problems faced by medical practitioners, such as the control of disease.

In learning disability, the use of scientific knowledge has been problematic. For example, its use has been seen by many as having contributed to the devaluing of people with learning disabilities because they have been compared to scientific constructs of what constitutes normality and, inevitably, have failed to measure up. Elsewhere, Marks-Maran (1999) warns against a reliance on scientific thinking to solve all of society's problems because it creates a culture in which anything that cannot be solved using scientific thinking is trivialised or dismissed. The emphasis on evidence based practice, for example, runs the risk of denigrating any practice that is not supported by a randomised controlled trial (Culshaw, 1995). Equally, as Parmenter (2001) points out, it would be wrong to assume that philosophy and values alone will bring about the lives that individuals want and that science could not provide some of the answers to problems.

Within learning disability nursing, the influence of this tension could be showing itself. For example, in interviews by Norman *et al.* (1996) some nurses expressed a frustration that they did not have a 'technology' to apply when working with individuals or a clearer framework on which to base their practice. A conference in 1996 (NHS Executive, 1996) on the issue of evidence based practice concluded that the use of scientifically derived evidence was underused within services because of a failure to manage knowledge successfully. The conference also concluded that the scientific knowledge base in learning disability was very low and tended to be related to specialist areas of practice such as challenging behaviour.

The message from this must be that effective practice should seek to integrate scientific knowledge with those aspects of practice that have been termed professional artistry. Within the practice chapters of this book, there are several examples to show how successful learning disability nurses could be at achieving this. Tim Riding, for example (see Chapter 2), uses O'Brien's (1987) five accomplishments as a framework for thinking about Alan's quality of life. The need to work in a person-centred way with Alan led Tim to use a self-control procedure based on evidence from cognitive behavioural interventions. Rebecca Welsh (see Chapter 12) also draws upon her specialist knowledge of epilepsy medication but she recognised the need to 'de-medicalise' this knowledge if she was going to work successfully with Tristan's mother. Finally, from one point of view, Colin Doyle's approach to working with Megan seems highly structured and based on learning theory (see Chapter 4). From another point of view, Colin was also conscious of the need to develop a relationship with Megan and her parents in order to effect positive change in their lives.

Generating knowledge from practice

In some instances, such as the examples given above, it is easy to identify the source of the knowledge used by nurses because it has been systematically generated, critically evaluated, published and made available to the professional community and others. The role of the practitioner then becomes one of seeking out knowledge that could be relevant to an issue or problem and then deciding how to apply this knowledge. In a way, this could be construed as a creative, or artistic endeavour. However, there are countless times when knowledge is not available to the learning disability nurse or it cannot solve the particular problem they face. For example, where was the research evidence that could have told Jackie Roberts (see Chapter 7) how to respond to Harry's mother's outburst in the hospital? What scientific evidence could Julie Wilkins (see Chapter 10) have used to help her respond positively to Jenna's relationships with the men on her residential unit?

The answer to these questions is that much of the knowledge that learning disability nurses need to be successful in their role is generated in the practice environment itself. If the aim of learning disability nursing is to help individuals with learning disabilities to construct a vision for their future, then this vision is more likely to be realised if the nurse is able to generate good quality information and knowledge from their encounter with the individual. The quality of information is first developed out of the relationship that the nurse has with the person and this is why the quality of the relationship between the nurse and the individual has become a major concern to nurses. In most studies into learning disability nursing, nurses have referred to the need to develop good relationships with service users and their families (Norman *et al.*, 1996; Alaszewski *et al.*, 2001). In spite of the importance of relationships, nurses have not described in detail their nature or how relationships should be managed.

Meutzel (1988) put forward a model for therapeutic relationships between nurses and clients comprising three elements of intimacy, partnership and reciprocity. This could form a useful starting point for defining the quality of relationships between nurses and individuals with learning disabilities. Despite the lack of a clear description, there are many examples from the practice chapters in this book which show how nurses have developed and managed their relationships that can be admired. Julie Wilkins (see Chapter 10) describes how she needed to help Jenna develop as a person and become more comfortable with herself. This meant that she would have to take a back seat on occasions. However, recognising this did not lessen the frustration. As Julie stated, 'It is sometimes very difficult to stand back and watch from a distance when your instincts are screaming at you to intervene'. Likewise, Jill Turner (see Chapter 3) recognised that disclosing information about herself could help develop her relationship with Sue, but she was careful not to disclose too much information.

As well as an emphasis on good quality relationships, another tool that enables nurses to generate useful knowledge from the practice environment is reflective practice. Whereas some have issued caution about the claims made for reflective practice (Burton, 2000), it has now become a central issue within nursing education, policy and practice where it is seen as an essential tool in promoting critical thinking and generating nursing theory (Boud *et al.*, 1998). According to Atkins & Murphy (1993) good reflection requires self-awareness, descriptive skills, the ability to formulate a problem or issue to be addressed, critical analysis, synthesising information and evaluation. Burrows (1995) commented how difficult it is to master the process of reflection and that it should be seen as being as skilful as the research process.

In relation to learning disability nursing Wolverson (2000) is in little doubt that learning disability nurses are not only skilled at reflection but are ahead of their other nursing colleagues. Wolverson adds that, in spite of their reflective skills, learning disability nurses do not often write about reflection or research into its use in their profession. Evidence from the practice examples in this chapter would suggest that all the contributors are highly reflective practitioners. Jill Turner (see Chapter 3) frames her entire chapter as a reflective account to demonstrate its value in helping her to work with Sue. However, of particular note is Jill's reflection on her own experience as a patient to develop her approach to working with people with learning disabilities. Julie Wilkins (see Chapter 10) also reports how she was caused to reflect when hearing herself deny Jenna the opportunity of going swimming without any real reason. Adrian Jones' (see Chapter 11) experience of supporting someone through a difficult time on his surgical ward led to him developing the determination to change the system from being 'service-centred' to 'person-centred'.

A moral purpose

Another key method that learning disability nurses employ to achieve their aims is to integrate ethical and moral principles into their decision-making. Reinders (1999) made the point that no amount of legislation and policy that set out the rights of people with learning disabilities is sufficient without people with the moral character to care. However, as Parmenter (2001) also commented, ethical principles should not be applied uncritically or seen as statements that have been formulated to prevent action. Instead, they are meant to act as a guide to help nurses and others to reflect on situations.

Published research studies in the field of learning disability nursing have not explicitly addressed how nurses use ethical principles in their decision-making. However, an unpublished study by Stanley *et al.* (1996) noted how ethical and moral principles are used by learning disability nurses as the key filter to appraise situations and events before acting upon them. Using critical incident analysis with nurses, the research team discovered that some of the main ethical principles that nurses considered before acting included the impact of events upon the safety of individuals, their autonomy, their right to freedom and to make choices.

The use of values and principles in decision-making features high on Moline's (1986) definition of professional practice. Moline includes values in his description of personal characteristics that he also uses to distinguish professionals from other workers. These characteristics add up to conveying a sense of responsibility and duty towards an individual. All the contributors to the practice chapters in this book convey a sense of calling and duty in their descriptions of how they came to be learning disability nurses. Their prime motivation seemed to be to work with people with learning disabilities rather than to be nurses which, it could be argued, gives them a strong sense of responsibility to people with learning disabilities. Managers in the Clifton *et al.* study (1992) reported that they admired nurses' professional attitude and sense of duty. Nurse respondents to Alaszewski *et al.* (2001) also listed personal characteristics as being a key component in their effectiveness as nurses. The practice chapters also list countless examples of where personal characteristics stand out as essential to the nurse's success. For example, Jackie Roberts (see Chapter 7) showed great patience and perseverance in the face of the anger and criticism of Harry's mother. In spite of events not always going as planned, Rebecca Welsh (see Chapter 12) also showed resolve in keeping up the spirits and the motivation of Tristan and his mother.

Final thoughts

This chapter set out to explore the aims of learning disability nursing practice and the decision-making processes that nurses use to work with individuals with learning disabilities. The sections have drawn attention to the importance of reflection, personal characteristics, the integration of scientific knowledge with aspects of professional artistry and the application of moral and ethical principles to practice situations. Although they have been described here as discrete elements of practice, it is probable that experienced nurses will synthesise these elements and ensure they are applied in a balanced way according to the demands of the situation. For example, in some situations the nurse will draw upon considerable scientific evidence, whereas in other situations the nurse will need to apply a greater amount of ethical or moral reasoning.

The profession has yet to develop a clear framework to explain how nurses use knowledge and make decisions about practice. However, Conway's (1998) investigation into expert nursing practice reveals similarities with learning disability nursing. For instance, Conway describes how expert nurses hold what she referred to as a 'world view' that comprised the values and philosophy of the nurse, the goals of the nurse, the reflective ability of the nurse and the resources available to them. Conway claimed that expert nurses could be distinguished by their ability to successfully integrate these elements and apply them in practice situations. Conway went on to describe four types of expert nurse that included 'technologists' who were nurses whose practice required them to apply technical and scientific knowledge. Another category included specialist nurses who, as the title suggests, worked in areas where they had extended their role. Conway also identified traditional expert practitioners whose expertise derived from managing resources well and getting things done. Finally, Conway gave the label 'humanistic existentialists' to nurses who saw themselves as responsible for developing the culture within practice environments.

The link may be tenuous at this stage but Conway's framework may have some resonance with the roles and ways of thinking about practice that have been developed by learning disability nurses. Perhaps, in due course, such a framework can be developed.

References

Alaszewski, A., Gates, B., Motherby, E., Manthorpe, J. & Ayer, S. (2001) *Educational preparation for learning disability nursing: outcomes evaluation of the contribution of learning disability nurses within the multi-professional, multi-agency team.* English National Board, London.

All Wales Nursing Group (1992) *A strategy for mental handicap nursing in Wales.* All Wales Nursing Group, Cardiff.

Atkins, S. & Murphy, K. (1993) Reflections: a review of the literature. *Journal of Advanced Nursing,* **18**, 735–40.

Barr, O. & Parahoo, K. (1994) A profile of learning disability nurses. *Nursing Standard,* 8(42), 35–9.

Birchenall, P. (1996) Learning disability nursing. Developing new horizons. *Nurse Education Today,* **16**, 83–4.

Blackmore, R. (2001) Advocacy in nursing. *Journal of Learning Disabilities,* **5**(3), 221–34.

Boud, D., Keough, R. & Walker, D. (1998) *Reflection: turning experience into learning.* Kogan Page, London.

Bradley, P. (1999) Perceptions of Health and Social Care Need – an exploratory study. *Learning Disability Practice,* **1**(3), 10–14.

Brown, J. (1994) *Analysis of responses to the consensus statement on the future of the specialist nurse practitioner in learning disabilities*. University of York, Department of Social Policy and Social Work, York.

Burrows, D. (1995) The nurse teacher's role in the promotion of reflective practice. *Nurse Education Today*, **15**(5), 24–8.

Burton, A.J. (2000) Reflection: nursing's practice and education panacea? *Journal of Advanced Nursing*, **31**(5), 1009–17.

Clifton, M., Shaw, I. & Brown, J. (1992) *Transferability of Mental Handicap Nursing Skills from Hospital to Community*. University of York Department of Social Policy and Social Work, York.

Conway, J.E. (1998) Evolution of the species 'expert nurse'. An examination of the practice knowledge held by expert nurses. *Journal of Clinical Nursing*, **7**, 75–82.

Culshaw, H. (1995) Evidence based practice for sale? *British Journal of Occupational Therapy*, **58**, 233.

Department of Health (1990) *NHS and Community Care Act*. HMSO, London.

Department of Health (1995) *Learning Disability: meeting needs through targeting skills*. Department of Health, London.

Department of Health and Social Security (1985) *The Role of the Nurse in Caring for People with Mental Handicap*, CNO (85)5. DHSS, London.

English National Board (1982) *Syllabus of training: professional register – part 5 (Registered Nurse for the Mentally Handicapped)*. English National Board, London.

English National Board (1985) *Education and Training of Nurses Caring for People with Mental Handicap*, Circular 1985/55ERDB. English National Board, London.

Four Chief Nursing Officers of The United Kingdom (1991) *Mental Handicap Nursing in the context of 'Caring for People'*. Department of Health, London.

Hall, V. & Russell, O. (1985a) Community mental handicap nursing – the birth, growth and development of the idea. In: Sines, D. & Bicknell, J. (eds) *Caring for Mentally Handicapped People in the Community*. Harper & Row, London.

Hall, V. & Russell, O. (1985b) Community Mental Handicap Nurses – their perceptions of what they do. In: Sines, D. & Bicknell, J. (eds) *Caring for Mentally Handicapped People in the Community*. Harper & Row, London.

Henderson, V. (1961) *Nature of Nursing*. Mosby, St. Louis.

Hunt, C., Wakefield, S. & Hunt, G. (2001) Community nurse learning disabilities: a case study of the use of an evidence-based screening tool to identify and meet the health needs of people with learning disabilities. *Journal of Learning Disabilities*, **5**(1), 9–18.

Kay, B., Rose, S. & Turnbull, J. (1995) *Continuing the Commitment: the report of the learning disability nursing project*. Department of Health, London.

Kerr, M., Fraser, W. & Felce, D. (1996) Primary healthcare for people with a learning disability. *British Journal of Learning Disabilities*, **24**(1), 2–8.

Leonard, A. (1988) *Out of Hospital. A survey of thirty centrally funded initiative schemes for children with mental handicaps*. University of York, York.

Marks-Maran, D. (1999) Reconstructing nursing: evidence, artistry and the curriculum. *Nurse Education Today*, **19**, 3–11.

Meutzel, P.A. (1988) Therapeutic nursing. In: Pearson, A. (ed) *Primary Nursing: nursing in the Burford and Oxford Nursing Development Units*. Croom Helm, Beckenham.

Mobbs, C., Hadley, S., Wittering, R. & Bailey, N.M. (2002) An exploration of the role of the community nurse, learning disability, in England. *British Journal of Learning Disabilities*, **30**, 13–18.

Moline, J. (1986) Professionals and professions: a philosophical examination of an ideal. *Social Science and Medicine*, **22**(5), 501–508.

National Health Service Executive (1996) *Clinical Effectiveness in Learning Disability*

Services: a report of an inter-agency seminar. November 7th. Anglia and Oxford NHS Executive Regional Office, Milton Keynes.

Norman, I., Redfern, S., Bodley, D., Holroyd, S., Smith, C. & White, E. (1996) *The Changing Educational Needs of Mental Health and Learning Disability Nurses.* English National Board, London.

O'Brien, J. (1987) A guide to lifestyle planning: using the activities catalogue to integrate services and natural support systems. In: Wilcox, B.W. & Bellamy, G.T. (eds) *The Activities Catalogue: an alternative curriculum for youth and adults with severe disabilities.* Brookes, Baltimore.

Parmenter, T.R. (2001) The contribution of science in facilitating the inclusion of people with intellectual disability into the community. *Journal of Intellectual Disability Research*, **45**(3), 183–93.

Raynes, N.V., Wright, K., Shiell A. & Pettipher, C. (1994) *The cost and quality of community residential care.* David Fulton Publishers, London.

Reinders, H.S. (1999) *Proceedings of the 10th World Congress of the International Association on the Scientific Study of Intellectual Disability.* IASSID, Washington, DC, USA.

Royal College of Nursing (1989) *Quality and Care – a strategy for Mental Handicap Nursing.* RCN, London.

Royal College of Nursing (1992) *The Role and Function of the Domiciliary Community Nurse for People with a Learning Disability.* RCN, London.

Royal College of Nursing (1994) *Learning Disability Nursing: an RCN guide for purchasers.* RCN, London.

Schon, D.A. (1987) *Educating the Reflective Practitioner.* Jossey-Bass, London.

Stanley, R., Boulter, P., Morritt, N., Gale, J. & Larner, J. (1996) *'Decision Making in the RNMH.' Unpublished Report for Learning Disability Nursing Project: host site initiative.* Lifecare NHS Trust, Coulsdon, Surrey.

Stewart, D. & Todd, M. (2001) Role and contribution of nurses for learning disabilities: a local study in a county of the Oxford-Anglia region. *British Journal of Learning Disabilities*, **29**, 145–50.

Turnbull, J. (1995) Services do need specialists. *Nursing Times*, **91**(49), 54.

United Kingdom Central Council (1987) *Project 2000. Working papers and final report.* UKCC, London.

Wolverson, M. (2000) On reflection. *Learning Disability Practice.* 3(2), 24–7.

Chapter 6

Lending an ear: helping someone to speak out

Peter Dawson

A student of life

When I was 20 I worked for a few months in a psychiatric hospital as a nursing assistant. I was constantly asked, by other members of staff, why I wasn't a student nurse. My stock reply was that I didn't really know what I wanted to do. One of my supportive colleagues replied for me once, saying, 'He is a student – a student of life!' Well, in one way that was true. I did learn something of life on those wards. I learned that the mostly old and confused men I tried to look after were worthy of more dignity and respect than the system of care was able to afford them. I learned that they were highly individual people with rich and varied pasts that were, at best, only obliquely hinted at by nurses but which nevertheless shone out of their sad or defiant eyes. I also came to the conclusion that I would never be a nurse.

Over the following six years I had a variety of work and life experiences. For instance, I lived and worked for 18 months in a community with people with learning disabilities. This was within a large voluntary organisation. The ethos there was such that everyone, regardless of impairment or role, was expected to participate in all the creative and cultural activities of the community. People with learning disabilities were valued in a way that made day-to-day life stimulating and largely satisfying.

Moving on, I lived and worked with children and young people with learning disabilities in a residential school in Sweden. This, too, was based on the Rudolf Steiner philosophy that had underpinned life in the community in England from which I had just come. The difference here was that workers were paid a living wage and the state ensured a high standard of basic provision.

By the mid 1970s, I was wondering where to go next. I had worked in a variety of situations besides working with people with learning disabilities. The vaguely hippie times I had embraced were coming to an end; I had family responsibilities and a growing desire to gain a qualification in something. Having been employed in shops and factories in my mid and late teens, I knew that I wanted to be with people rather than products and that I liked people with learning disabilities. I suppose I also had an unclear but strong notion that I wanted to do something useful. Someone I knew suggested that I should enquire about training as a nurse in the local mental handicap hospital, as it was called then, and, before I could say 'Jack Robinson', I was signed up for a three-year course. This was despite my absolute conviction five years earlier that I would never do that. The plain facts were that I now wanted a career and some security working with people whose company I thought I would enjoy. Another factor in choosing a nursing career was that, as far as I could see, no other course of training existed that would equip and qualify me to work specifically with people with learning disabilities. Somewhere within this mixture of motives was the belief that I could make a difference.

Bleak surroundings

The first ward on which I was placed during my training provided me with something of a culture shock. There were severely disabled men lying around on the floor in various states of continence and clothing.

'What we do here,' the charge nurse told me, 'is put food in one end and mop it up at the other.'

I crouched down on the floor and started talking to the men there. I was swiftly beckoned back to the wall.

'No point in doing that,' I was told, 'they don't understand.'

It would be nice if I could say, with hand on heart, that from the beginning I bucked the trend and treated everyone I met with equal respect, dignity and value. But in any strong institution there is pressure to conform. I drew as much as I could on my inner knowledge and past experience but my stance was generally interpreted as naive or uninformed. I suspect that there were a considerable number of people in nursing at that time who really wanted to change things but, like me, didn't really know how. It seemed to be a matter of hanging in there and attempting to infiltrate people's attitudes with the best principles and practices of nursing that were available.

After qualifying I was soon promoted to charge nurse and for the following six years I managed wards at the hospital as well as taking a secondment, for six months, as an unqualified nurse tutor. Wolfensberger's normalisation theory (1972) was starting to have an impact nationally and hospital managers became resentfully aware that institutional provision might have to change. Psychological approaches were also challenging the traditional power base of psychiatry within the service. Because of this, behaviour modification techniques, room management (Jenkins *et al.*, 1987) and regular ward reviews began to be used. I welcomed these innovations, sometimes with slight scepticism about whether they controlled people with learning disabilities, but on the whole hopeful that the lives of people with learning disabilities would improve.

Improving my knowledge and understanding was still a personal quest. A course I found eye-opening was the Open University's 'The Handicapped Person in the Community'. This was good for a number of reasons, the main one being that it introduced me to the social model of disability. I had often felt that people with learning disabilities, especially those with challenging behaviours, were blamed for their impairment. Suddenly, I had a theoretical model that explained a view that people with impairment were in a social and historical context that disabled them through institutional structures and attitudes. This made a lot of sense but still didn't give me a name for the way I wanted to work with people.

A spirited character

I met Judith in what turned out to be my final role at the hospital – my appointment as manager of the social skills unit. Judith was looking for a different life, but only half-heartedly. She came three days a week to the unit that was situated in a large, detached house on the edge of the hospital grounds, trudging and swearing her way along the half mile from her ward. She was clearly fed up and saw coming to the house as a chance to sit and smoke and to have a change of scenery. Her mantra was 'I want to leave this f...ing dump!' By this she meant the hospital, but her general demeanour and the lack of hope in her eyes spelt out that she did not believe it could happen.

At this time Judith was approaching her mid-forties. She was a well-built woman with a shock of blonde hair and a ruddy complexion. The tight and rather short print dresses she wore did her figure no favours and her cheap and garish cardigans were often inside out. She did not care much about her appearance. Judith was on a daily programme of independence training but she did not enjoy the company of the other women with whom she was expected to train. Instead of the cleaning and cooking that was part of her programme Judith spent as much time as she could sighing and swearing and, when in a good mood, chatting to staff (preferably men). Despite her boredom and general apathy it was considered, from occasional displays of talent, that Judith was very capable of many self-help tasks. Comments about local or national news and insightful contributions to hospital gossip also confirmed that, beneath her brooding presence, there was a spirited individuality and intelligence. Judith was thought of as a character on the wards. She was known to play the clown, pull funny faces at times and to go for days without speaking when she 'had a bag on!'

Over the following weeks she disguised her lack of numeracy and literacy skills quite well but I did eventually suspect that she had very little of either. Though she was said to be unexpectedly generous and witty on occasion, she was introduced to me principally as someone who needed watching. She had a reputation for flaring up violently when asked to do something that she didn't want to do. She was on a regular small dose of tranquillisers and her slight but constant shake was fairly certainly a side effect of this.

A sympathetic ear

To be honest, I greatly sympathised with her lack of commitment to house cleaning and did not, in any case, see that as being the be-all and end-all of social training. Judith came to the training house three times a week. I was not always there as I often had meetings to attend or visits to make. But I had not long been in my appointment before she would be bringing me luke-warm cups of tea at regular intervals whenever I was in the building. Sitting nearby, often out of direct eye contact at first, she began to tell me her life story, or at least as much of it as she wanted me to know. Her speech was punctuated with colourful expletives but the gist was this: she had been born and brought up in the rough end of a Midlands city. Her mother was on the game.

'Do you know what shagging means, Peter?'

I got the start of this story several times until she felt she could move on. I would confirm that I understood but she would continue by saying,

'It's screwing men for money. Did you know that?'

After some weeks of telling me this, other bits of history came out. She had been brought to the hospital at the age of 16.

'It was tough in them days. We had to clean the floor in rows: all of us bent down with cloths and polishing with nurse standing over us telling us to get on with it.'

After a year or two at that she was sent to the hospital's hostel eight miles away in the town.

'It was all right there at first. The other girls started to get on my wick, though. I was always in trouble for fighting and being cheeky to the staff.'

She was there for a total of 16 years and was eventually returned to the hospital. No explanation was given. Judith's version is that 'they was probably fed up with me!'

I had this account in bits and pieces over several weeks. Then one day she suddenly said,

'I had a baby.'

'Where?' I asked, taken by surprise.

'At the hostel?'

'No, not bloody there: a long time ago when I was with my mam in the city. That's why I came in here in the first place!'

I was not surprised or shocked. I was interested and also touched for as she told me her eyes filled with tears.

'They took it away!'

'Was it a boy or a girl?' I asked.

'Dunno,' she replied, 'can't remember.'

It is at times like that that you get an inkling of the overwhelming sadness of people's lives. Judith, as far as many other people were concerned, was the often belligerent but also comic and sometimes saucy character everyone thought they knew. I had been privileged to see a deeper side.

'Any road,' she would say after a particularly intense conversation, 'I want to get out of this f…ing dump.'

I talked to her sometimes about what she liked and disliked about living in the hospital. She was quite clear that it was not where she wanted to live. She repeated frequently, and often without swearing, that she wanted to live on her own, in a flat in town. She was quite sure that she would manage on her own. I totally believed her desire for independence but there was an element of doubt in my mind as to her capabilities. I had never seen her sustain any daily living skills activity for more than a few minutes. She soon got bored and restless with the routines that were part of her programme. She did, however, have an immensely well-tuned sensitivity. If I was feeling harassed or having trouble of some kind she immediately picked up the vibe and would ask me what was up.

'Go on, you can tell me,' she'd say. 'I'm not going to tell any bugger!'

So, amongst the other bits of conversation we had she was allowing me to emerge as a person as well as a manager or nurse and I was allowing myself to relate to her as a person first and a patient, client, or whatever, second. At the bottom of all this was a sense of two people listening to each other and valuing what they heard.

I mentioned to colleagues that Judith was expressing a strong desire to leave the hospital and manage on her own. Generally they 'pooh-poohed' her idea saying that it would be irresponsible to let her go. This view seemed largely based on a notion of Judith as a dangerous sexual entity who would spend all her time seducing strangers and would set up some sort of 'knocking shop' in her accommodation. I was extremely doubtful of this. What she said that she wanted more than anything was a quiet life, on her own, away from all the other girls and bossy staff.

'You know, she had a baby? It's in her notes!' I was told by the unit's staff nurse. I replied that yes, I did know, as she had told me herself.

'Ah, you're just a soft touch,' the staff nurse continued, 'She's after anything in trousers!'

I failed to see how having a baby nearly 30 years previously meant that she was sexually promiscuous now. In any case, what sort of judgement were we making even if she was?

A twist in the tale

What occurred next, however, brought a new twist to this story and to our relationship. I was soon to take up a different job. After nine years of working at the hospital my own discharge was looming! The post was a joint finance appointment between the health authority and social services, working with the local social services on a senior social work level as a coordinator of Individual Programme Planning (IPP).

One evening in my last month at the unit Judith stopped me on my way out of the building.

'I want to see you Peter,' she said. 'It's important and private!'

We found a quiet space. I sensed that this was something extra to our usual chats.

'You must promise not to tell anyone,' she insisted.

I agreed. She got straight to the point.

'I'm doing it,' she informed me. And just in case I had doubts as to her meaning, she added, 'with Jim – we're screwing.'

I enquired gently as to why she was telling me this.

'Well aren't you shocked?' she demanded. I shook my head.

'Where are you "doing it"?'

'Under the bushes outside the kitchens,' was the reply.

'Why there?' I enquired.

'Come on Peter, you're not that bloody daft are you? If *they* knew what we were doing Jim would be in the locked ward and I'd be in a right load of trouble with the doctor.' This was true. I asked her what she thought of having sex with Jim.

'It's all right,' she mused. 'It's what he wants really. He's all right. He's nice.' Jim was a patient on one of the men's blocks. He was a rugged and quietly spoken man. I was surprised but immediately recognised that I was perhaps naive to be surprised. Jim was quite a gentle character, about Judith's own age. Nobody would have obviously linked them together. But they had known each other a long time.

I felt sad at the thought of these two people who both had a natural dignity, feeling forced to express themselves sexually in the dirt, like animals. I was also confused. On one hand what Judith was telling me could be thought to confirm what others had said about her sexual behaviour. I felt, however, that it confirmed her desperation and her need for a dignified life outside the confines of the hospital.

'Anyway,' she continued, 'I'm doing it. We often do it, me and Jim. We like it. It's all right. He treats me like a lady.'

Further confusion. Did she really enjoy sex with Jim? Why was she telling me all this. I asked her again.

'Because I'm scared,' she said.

'Scared of being found out?' I asked.

'No. Scared of having a baby.'

Ah, so that was it. I thought about Judith's age.

'Bit old for a baby?'

'My mam was old when she had me,' she answered.

I felt out of my depth. Then I remembered that she was on the pill. I reminded her of this and she asked,

'What's the pill?'

Inwardly I sighed in exasperation that nobody had taken time out to explain to her about that certain pill she took regularly. I talked a bit about it and told her I would find out more. We also talked about her 'doing it' on the ground and how that might not be the most comfortable place. She seemed unconcerned about this, saying that she didn't mind where she 'did it' providing Jim was happy and she didn't have a baby. We ended our conversation with me reaffirming, on her demand, that I would not tell anybody what she was doing. I felt uneasy, but also quite certain that I was the only person besides herself and Jim, and possibly one or two other observant patients, who knew. I decided to gather information for her about contraception and also to find out ways to check out her rights to sexual fulfilment in comfortable surroundings.

Two or three days later, however, she told me.

'I'm in trouble, I can't see Jim any more. I'm not allowed out except with a nurse.'

I asked her what had happened. She confessed that the day before she had decided, presumably having plucked up courage from our conversation, to tell the staff nurse on the unit about her sex life. The nurse had immediately reported the whole matter to the consultant. He, in turn, had put restrictions in place to prevent Judith and Jim from meeting together unsupervised.

'I didn't say anything,' I assured her.

'I know you didn't.'

But I felt a sick feeling and I felt confused. Should I have shared Judith's disclosure? Should I have acted more quickly and got back to her with information about the pill? In hindsight whatever I had done or not done would, I suspect, have resulted in the same effect. In other words, sex was not allowed between patients and that any person with a learning disability indulging in sex would be likely to be punished. But why on earth was Judith on the pill anyway if she was not allowed sex?

Being hauled up in front of the consultant and reprimanded had initially made Judith embarrassed and quite aggressive to anyone who stepped in her way. For the next few weeks she was escorted to and from the unit by a nurse from her ward. I decided to take matters into my own hands and so wrote to the consultant asking for clarity about patients' sexual freedoms. I got a letter back that was obscure and made reference to 'crown property' and legislation, that was unspecified, that forbade anybody from having sexual intercourse on hospital property. I thought wryly about the two nurses who were known to use the linen cupboard regularly on one particular ward. I decided not to pursue that line. It must have been about this time that the same consultant sent me a copy of a letter he had written to the health authority complaining that he had never, in all his professional life, been so insulted by having to justify his decisions to a mere underling such as me. I don't think he got a reply. At least, if he did I never saw it.

Eventually, some of Judith's routines were resumed. She was allowed through the hospital grounds again without escort to go to the social skills unit but she was carefully watched the rest of the time. Just before leaving the job, to move on into the joint funded post I was taking up, we had a last long talk. She was just as fed up as ever, frustrated, I think, at not being allowed to be her own person. Judith was accepting of her lot in certain ways. For example, about the incident under the bush, she said,

'Well, I shouldn't have bloody done it I suppose. I got what I deserved.'

However, she was still as adamant as ever that she wanted to leave the hospital and live on her own 'in my own little flat, somewhere in town'. I took note but made no promises to her. I remember saying,

'Well, if you get your own place you'll be able to have sex comfortably!'

'Fat chance of that,' or words to that effect, was her reply as she slouched away to cadge a cigarette or make a cuppa.

As I watched her and saw what she had been reduced to by the institution, I knew that she was, inside, a total person, a woman with dignity and wit and warmth, who deserved the existence she craved which was, in fact, only an ordinary life.

New opportunities

I was soon making a few interesting discoveries in my new job. Though I was appointed as a senior social worker, I found it easy to use my nursing knowledge and skills. This presented challenges to me and my new professional colleagues and the first few months of my job were spent in proving to them that I was indeed capable of doing the job, part of which was supervising social services staff. A large element of my role was identifying and supporting residents of the hospital to leave and live in the community, with appropriate support networks. To me, the attraction, strength and advantage of this, the Individual Programme Planning (IPP) was that the person whose plan it was would be in the central role determining the process and outcome of the plan.

It was for this reason that I got back in touch with Judith. Some months had gone by. My life had changed dramatically: a new place of work, different colleagues and new personal objectives. Judith's life had not changed. I quickly checked with her that she still wanted to leave the hospital. I explained my new job and said that I would be able to help her leave the hospital. I could arrange for her to get her own place with support staff who would help her manage day to day. She was extremely doubtful that any of this would happen.

'They won't let me', she repeated. 'And, anyway, I wouldn't need any help in the house if I did move. They'd only be spies for the hospital!'

I foresaw a few problems in planning a service for Judith that would be acceptable to everyone concerned. But I kept those thoughts to myself, remaining positive. Judith agreed to give it a shot, so, in accordance with the principles of good practice, I asked her who she would want at her first IPP meeting. She wasn't sure about this.

'Can't we just do it through chatting, you and me?' she asked.

I felt my hands were tied and explained that she was more likely to be able to leave the hospital if a group of people she liked and trusted, who knew her well, got together and planned things from the start. She identified a couple of people who she thought were important which were the staff nurse on the unit and the junior consultant psychiatrist. We set a date and time for her first meeting. I arranged with her for someone to see her from my new team in order to start working with her and to get to know her a little. I booked the sitting room in the social skills unit and went away in the hope that everything would fall into place. We had three or four weeks to plan the first meeting and get our act together.

The morning of the first meeting arrived and I had received, in advance, encouraging reports from my team's worker that she and Judith were getting on well and that Judith was enjoying the individual attention. They had been around town together a few times and Julie, the team member, had taken Judith home with her once or twice for cups of tea or snacks. Together they had even started to talk about the sort of flat she might like to live in in the future. But that had only been in the most vague of terms and the point of the early contact had really been to support Judith to feel that we were serious about helping her to get out and live a more independent life. The object of our first proper IPP meeting was to formalise this. By having Judith in the central position within the meeting I wanted to emphasise that this was her life, her future and that she had a right and the ability to play a part in determining what was going to happen.

A spanner in the works

What do they say about the best-laid plans of mice and men? The first problem was hit just ten minutes before the meeting was due to start. The nursing officer in charge of the unit, who six months earlier had been my own supportive boss, turned up demanding to be part of the meeting. She had not been invited as Judith found her generally to be rather intimidating. I now realise that I was not assertive enough to say 'no', so into the meeting she went. She then sat bristling in a corner, muttering that the IPP scheme was only in existence to criticise 30 years of loving care towards difficult 'subnormals' who would otherwise, and still could be, homeless on the street.

By the time Judith arrived the unit's staff nurse, who thought it wise to be in league with her nursing officer, had insisted that a student nurse unknown to either Judith or myself also sat in on the meeting. The junior consultant arrived late with his pager buzzing. The only person I felt any confidence in was Julie, who had gone for a coffee with Judith before the meeting and who bounced in with notes she had made to support Judith's strategy over the next few weeks. What the meeting was in danger of becoming right from the outset was some sort of discharge tribunal rather than a planning group. Was this a problem that I had caused as convenor of the meeting?

My own strategy was to work from the basis that we all agreed that Judith was leaving the hospital and that the scheme which I coordinated would facilitate that. But the gathering rapidly slipped away from such laudable objectives. The nursing officer was soon saying in a very powerful manner that the social service's proposal that Judith left the hospital was extremely irresponsible and that I should know better, having worked with Judith, than to think that there was any way she could live on her own. The consultant said, to Judith's face,

'In any case she won't want to leave here, even if you give her the chance. She just won't want to!'

I tried to remind the meeting that this was Judith's meeting and that she was here amongst us and that her wishes should be listened to. I asked her what she wanted to do and she was brave enough to say, in a timid voice that she *did* want to leave the hospital and live on her own.

It was a few minutes after that that Judith left the room. She was in tears at the bullying and negativity that she was encountering. Julie followed her out. She, too, had felt intimidated and close to tears. I closed the meeting officially but reiterated that the scheme which Judith was embarking on was one which would ensure appropriate support to her, in the community. I explained that we would continue getting to know Judith and find out what her needs were, that we would liaise with staff. Most of this seemed to fall on stony ground but I assured those present that I would reconvene the meeting in a few weeks time. The hospital staff went away shaking their heads and muttering, 'It won't work.' I knew for Judith's sake it had to, but how?

Basically we kept in there! Another few weeks went by. Julie, whom I supervised, continued to work with Judith and to keep me informed. They were obviously getting on well and this showed itself in Judith's general appearance and motivation and, unexpectedly, in her language. I also talked to Judith myself, reassuring her that we really were getting somewhere. One thing we had discovered was that she was not as familiar with ovens and cooking equipment as had previously been assumed. The cups of tea she frequently delivered to all and sundry had probably been made earlier by other people. In other words her skills were not great, or at least the motivation to demonstrate or improve them was not. Julie began to increase Judith's time in social training and to provide her with one-to-one tuition from her own team of home care aides.

By the next meeting things were starting to take shape. We were now armed with a plan outlining Judith's needs for support and her wants with regard to accommodation. The psychiatrist sent his apologies. Judith and Julie and one of the home care aides were all there, as was the staff nurse from the unit. For reasons that she did not justify, the nursing officer stayed away from the meeting even though I had invited her, with Judith's agreement. However, an occupational therapist and psychologist had joined the group.

We were now at the point in the scheme where we could put in a request to a housing association for a flat for Judith. We could also start to cost out what support she would need from our service. Judith was not at all happy about the prospect of having people come in to what would be her new home. She repeated that she could look after herself and didn't need anybody snooping on her and making her do stuff. Julie gently reminded her that there were things she would need help with at the start but that she would be able to do those things for herself with practice. The staff nurse, however, whilst disagreeing that Judith needed help to look after herself practically was firmly of the opinion that she would be isolated and at risk of loneliness and generally vulnerable on her own in a flat. In between the first and second meeting I had worked on my own confidence and style of delivery and felt that the meeting was going well and that this time conflict was being handled appropriately. I was chairing the meeting again and one major thing I had managed to ensure was that Judith was addressed rather than being spoken about in the third person.

It was at this point, when the winning post was in sight, that the hospital played its trump card. The psychologist said that she had interviewed Judith and that she was strongly of the opinion that Judith ought to move into a shared flat rather than live on her own. Judith declared vehemently that this was not what she wanted and once again the meeting ended on a sour note. The staff nurse said that he would talk to her and the meeting ended. As far as I was concerned we had the brief from Judith to find single accommodation. We would arrange the support she needed to live in it. The home care aide team who had been working with her would continue to do so prior to us finding her a suitable flat. They would also be able to provide her with support once she had left the hospital. In effect the meeting had concluded inconclusively.

A setback

After this, things took further unexpected and dramatic turns. I had been away on a course and it was not until a fortnight after the meeting I heard what had happened. Julie rang me to say that Judith was now on the locked ward at the hospital, having hit other residents, putting one of them in casualty. I gradually pieced the story together. The staff nurse had persuaded Judith to consider living in a shared apartment. His argument was that Judith could not make up her mind without trying it! To this end he had arranged, very suddenly, for Judith to go and stay with a woman she had been friendly with two or three years previously when they had both lived at the hostel. Judith's erstwhile friend was now in a small flat on the outskirts of town; an area Judith was not familiar with.

The arrangements seemed to have been made hastily and without reference to anyone within social services. The staff nurse took Judith to the other woman's flat and provided a camp bed for Judith to sleep in. Looking back I think the staff nurse was acting in order to prove a point he strongly believed in, and with the best of intentions, but without having really listened to Judith. We were all in danger of taking entrenched positions without really believing in what Judith said and finding out the best way to achieve what she wanted.

After two uneasy nights under the same roof as her friend Judith had come back to the hospital, using public transport on her own initiative. The trial had failed in as much as she had argued with her friend and had not stuck it out for the whole weekend. On the other hand she had, of course, been saying all along that she did not want to share! So she had come back to the unit. Two of the other residents, who Judith had never got on with, made scathing and irritating remarks about her failure and, hey presto, Judith had flown off the handle and given them both 'a bit of fist'. One was unhurt but the other had a cut to her nose and a blow to her forehead that required a stitch. Judith herself, angry and distraught had run the distance between the unit and the hospital and reported what she had done.

It was hardly the crime of the century and I strongly suspect she was provoked. Indeed, the whole of the abrupt arrangement, that she had not wanted, could be considered a provocation. Unfortunately, by acting as she had she was proving the wrong people right. And however well I justified to myself the process to this point I felt guilty that it was going so horribly wrong. Judith deserved better support than this. I went as quickly as I could to the hospital and sought out her ward. I was let on and Judith looking defiant greeted me.

'That's it then Peter. You did your best.'

'Do you still want to leave?' I asked her.

She told me that she was fed up of messing about and not getting anywhere.

'Get me out in three months or I'll stay here forever!'

She had given me one more chance to help her and an ultimatum. Shortly after that we had a team meeting and we all agreed that we had to pull out the stops.

This took slightly less than three months. As soon as we had a place for Judith to move into I decided to call a final IPP meeting. Prior to this Julie and her team resumed contact with Judith. She had not gone back to the unit and so we were by now liaising with her ward staff. At least Judith was back on her regular ward as opposed to the locked one. Julie and her team had worked hard with Judith to help her to get to know the area and to familiarise herself with her, soon to be, new abode. Together they had chosen, bought and cadged fixtures, fittings and furniture.

Our meeting this time comprised the ward sister, who I had spent some time talking to about Judith's plans, the junior consultant, the community nurse who would be keeping an eye on Judith, Julie and one member of her team. I had encouraged Judith to bring a friend to the meeting and she had in fact invited the woman with whom she had fallen out a few weeks earlier in the flat in town. The two of them sat together and I realised that Judith had been quite clever. The other woman was friendly and quite pleased to be asked to the meeting but did confirm without hesitation that Judith would be far better off in a flat of her own! The upshot of this final, hospital-based meeting was that Judith was able to announce that she now had the keys to her own flat and that she would be moving in within the following ten days. Arrangements were made, with her reluctant agreement, that home care aides would call three times a day and stay up to two hours, helping her to clean and shop and sort out bills. Night cover was also briefly mooted by the hospital staff but quickly dismissed by Judith with my backing. People wished her well and there did seem to have been a turnaround of feeling about her moving out. I'm sure that secretly the doctor did not believe she would go and that he was right all along in saying she did not want to – but at least he now had the courtesy to give her the benefit of the doubt.

On the move

The move itself went brilliantly. Judith's flat was in a new block in a housing association complex with a common room downstairs. A warden was on call and had soon got to know Judith. We scheduled a review of the arrangements for a month after Judith had got in. I went around to see her. Julie was there and the community nurse. Judith had also invited Marion, one of the home helps, who had taken a shine to her, to join in. Judith made us a pot of tea, which was hot. She also produced a packet of biscuits and settled back in her comfy sofa, fag in one hand and ashtray in the other. The meeting was informal and it was abundantly clear that she was, at last, happy with her life.

'Don't mind if I watch this film duck, do you?' she asked.

She did, however, show me around her domain with pride, before I got the hint and we left her in peace. The daily support she initially got from our scheme had rapidly reduced. This was by her own request and also from Julie's assessment that Judith was now showing that she could manage most things on her own. As I left her flat I had caught, out of the corner of my eye, the shine of ornaments on her shelf, over the gas fire.

'They're new,' she told me with pride: a dog, a cat and two other figures. I asked her as we departed whether she was happy for us to hold the occasional meeting with her in her house to make sure everything was going according to plan. No, she said. No more meetings. However, after a pause, she added

'but you can have a get together now and then, if you want'.

Some weeks later I called in one day as I was nearby. She was pleased to see me but preoccupied, dusting the now several shelves of shining porcelain ornaments. These were immaculately kept and I had never seen her so industrious.

'I call them my babies,' she muttered.

She was looking well and her medication had been reduced. Despite still having a slight wobble the care she lavished on her 'babies' was such that none would fall from her firm grasp as she dusted and polished each one individually. That proved to be the last time I spoke to her as new organisational arrangements meant that her IPP was transferred from my coordination to that of a colleague. We were able, however, to make sure that she had the same domicilary team working with her and it was from them that I got regular updates about her progress over the following years.

At first Judith spent regular Saturday or Sunday afternoons back at the hospital. She missed the company of the women with whom she had got so bored previously. After a while, though, these visits reduced. Her collection of ornaments, however, grew to the point where it would have been a case of Judith having to find another place to live and keeping her flat on as an extended china cupboard! Fortunately she was persuaded to see the sense of cutting back on the collection. The fears that had been voiced about her promiscuity were far from realised. In fact, a neighbour who she had known years before at the hospital made advances to her which were rebuffed in no uncertain terms. Her care hours continued to be reduced on her request until she was only receiving one visit a day. She was reputed to be putting on weight to a large degree due to a daily penchant for chips. She was still a heavy smoker. The community nurse had a good relationship with her. She seemed to understand risks to her health but it was her life and she would now live it how she wanted.

End of the road

After the first couple of years the most surprising thing of all was her social life. Judith had eventually abandoned the housing association common room in favour of the church and its hall across the road. This was a Catholic church and I had not known of any associations that Judith had ever had with that faith. She became a regular attender and developed an unexpected friendship with a fellow parishioner. He was an elderly, retired solicitor. They were constantly in each other's company and developed a genuine and deep affection and appreciation of each other. After a couple of years he contracted a terminal illness and she was a devoted visitor at his bedside. She grieved at his death and never replaced him in her affections. His family had found it hard to understand why he had taken to this sometimes rather surly and overweight woman with a learning disability. I don't. She was insightful and warm and had a gentleness that she was prepared to show abundantly to those who were gentle with her.

About two years after her friend died Judith also passed away. She had been out of the hospital for about ten years by this time. I had last caught a glimpse of her about a year before she died. I had seen her in the distance, struggling on foot up a long hill in the centre of town. She was very large and was carrying two shopping bags, with a determined look on her face. She could have been any working woman, mother or grandmother on her way home. How many more years of freedom might she have enjoyed had she been listened to earlier? How many other people might have benefited from her as a fellow citizen?

Final thoughts

There are other people I could have written this chapter about – people I knew better or worked with for longer, or more recently. There are a couple of reasons why I chose to write about Judith. One is that the way I tried to work with her, however inadequately, was through her self-advocacy and towards an objective of empowerment. These are not words that were in my use 17 years ago when we first met. Empowerment is the name I sought back then for the model I was attempting to identify. Self-advocacy is the tool. Judith taught me an invaluable lesson and set me on a path from which I could never turn back.

The lesson is that our duty as nurses, or just people working with people with learning disabilities, is to recognise and work to the authority of *their* direct experience. Only they know what it is like to be people with learning disabilities subjected to the services other people decree for them. They are the experts. Nurses are often in a good position to support people to develop and use the voice to say effectively what their lives are like and what it is they want. The approach of the nurse is practical as well as value based. Nurses should have the values of empowerment and self-advocacy in heart as well as head. They can help to make things happen. If, however, they are working with people who are already using their voice it is inexcusable not to listen.

References

Jenkins, J., Felce, D., Mansell, J., de Kock, U. & Toogood, S. (1987) Organising a residential service. In: Yule, W. & Carr, J. (eds) *Behaviour Modification for People with Mental Handicaps*. Croom Helm, London.

Wolfensberger, W. (1972) *The Principle of Normalisation in Human Services*. NIMH, Toronto.

Chapter 7

A new start: earning the trust of a family

Jackie Roberts

A nervous start

The road to self-discovery is a long one with many peaks and troughs. My journey to becoming the nurse I am today started when I was 19. I was training to be a nursery nurse and in my second year at college. I vividly remember being sent to a special school in a remote area. I was told that it was an opportunity to work with handicapped children. I had no knowledge or experience of children with a handicap and so I had no idea of what to expect. I can recall feeling nervous, apprehensive and not sleeping particularly well the evening before. I arrived at the school early the following morning, where a rather grave woman stepped out to meet me. I didn't dare ask who she was and she was definitely not going to introduce herself.

The first ten minutes, whilst waiting for everyone to arrive, felt like hours. It was agonising, to say the least. I remember wondering whether I would make it through the day as I felt nauseous and vulnerable. Then, out of the blue, a young woman with a bright beaming smile and chirpy voice said,

'Hi, would you be Jackie? I'm Sue, welcome,' and she vigorously shook my hand. On uttering 'yes', I felt an overwhelming sense of relief. It was as if a heavy boulder had been lifted off my shoulders and I felt safe again. As it happened, I thoroughly enjoyed my placement at the school. In fact, I enjoyed it so much that I volunteered to go on the school holiday. It was only at the end of the course that I realised that my time at the special school was only the beginning of a never-ending journey.

I began my nurse training shortly after qualifying as a nursery nurse. I don't think that I knew at the time whether I wanted to be a nurse, but I did know that I needed to find out who handicapped adults were. My perception of handicapped adults was so very different to the reality that I was about to encounter. I suddenly found myself enveloped in a very unfamiliar culture. It was alien to my values on life and experiences of communicating with people. I found myself being spoken to and told to do, what at the time, seemed hideous acts. There are too many to recount but a couple in particular stand at the forefront of my memory.

I had not been in placement for many weeks and the days were long. It soon, however, became apparent that at three o'clock every afternoon everyone, regardless of whether they wanted one or not, was given a cup of tea out of a huge kettle-like pot. The tea was mixed with milk and sugar. I didn't see this activity as groundbreaking nursing intervention and decided one afternoon to take the initiative to make the tea. After all, there was nothing else to do. I began handing the tea out to the elderly ladies and gentlemen, feeling quite pleased that I had carried out such a simple task without being told to do so, when a loud, deep voice boomed from the other side of the day room.

'Who told you to make the tea?' I recall being asked.

'No one', I replied.

'I didn't tell you to make the tea did I?' was the response from the nurse.

She then retrieved the tea from those I had given it to and tipped it back into the large teapot. I was then told to go and make the tea again because I was only to do things when told to. I was completely and utterly baffled by the nurse's response to my actions. I had never been treated in such a derogatory manner. I was stunned and puzzled.

That evening I thought long and hard about my day and I asked myself whether I should continue with the training. I found, much to my amazement an incredible urge of determination to carry on, as I knew I had an obligation to the patients. I also knew that I had an enormous challenge to stand up to being controlled. The road from there on was quite rough and bumpy. There were only a few smooth passages before I qualified.

From the outset of my nurse training I felt that I had strong beliefs about how people with a learning disability should be treated. After all, in less than one year I had experienced what felt like considerable oppression and marginalisation myself. I questioned internally how it must feel to spend one's life at the mercy of others, to have to wake up when told, to eat when told and not to be able to wear clothes that were mine.

I also found, much to my surprise that my journey to becoming a learning disability nurse was nothing like I had imagined it to be. I had assumed from the outset that to be a learning disability nurse it was necessary to care. However, my training just taught me to follow instructions and to comply with a system. I vividly recall watching a young woman being taken from a ward and put into the back of a minibus. She was taken to a hostel, which was to be her new home. I felt guilt, shame and pity as I watched her leave. She had absolutely no idea where she was going and I felt powerless to intervene.

My training was, without doubt, a test. It taught me a great deal about myself. It taught me the importance of self-acceptance; to be confident about what I believed in and to accept others for who they are. It taught me about resilience and integrity.

First encounter with Harry

It was a bleak winter's day when I first met Harry. I had received the referral a couple of days before I arranged to meet him. The referral requested that Harry should receive support to move from the hospital where he was convalescing to a residential home a couple of miles away. Harry had sustained a fracture to his tibia bone and had been in hospital for almost five months. Prior to his hospitalisation Harry had lived with his parents. It was felt by the medical team that provision should be made for Harry to transfer within the next four weeks, as he had made satisfactory progress. I had received information from my manager that the care manager had been in contact with Harry's parents who had discussed with them the suitability of the move and that the parents were happy with the decision. The care manager was now requesting a health profile to pass on to those staff that would be supporting Harry.

It was my responsibility to collate the data in order that up-to-date information about Harry's health could be passed on. I considered the referral to be relatively straightforward. I arranged a time to meet with the named nurse supporting Harry and to meet Harry as well. I arrived at the ward where Harry was residing. It appeared very busy and I observed many elderly people there. I had quite a wait until the nurse was available. There was a strong odour of stale urine, which lingered in the ward, and staff seemed to be in a frenetic state, attending to the constant requests from the elderly patients. After approximately 15 minutes I was greeted by a young female nurse and I introduced myself. The nurse was welcoming and briefly explained Harry's progress to date. I asked if it would be possible to meet Harry in order that I could make him aware of my involvement. The nurse agreed and I was taken to Harry's bed.

Harry was preoccupied with some books when I arrived at his bedside. He slowly raised his head and looked astounded as I stood there with the nurse. The nurse introduced me by saying,

'Harry, this is Jackie – she's a new nurse who's going to help you with your move to your new home.'

At this, the nurse excused herself and I was left with Harry. I said hello to Harry and asked him how he was. There was an immediate look of bewilderment on Harry's face when I asked him this.

'Who are you?' was the response.

'I'm Jackie – I'm a nurse from the learning disability team.'

On reflection, I could have told Harry that I was the Queen of Sheba because he seemed to have no concept of who or what a learning disability nurse was. I had an immediate sinking feeling as Harry lowered his head and continued to flick through his books.

'I would like to see you again Harry – is that okay?'

'Yes,' was Harry's reply. I said goodbye and notified Harry's named nurse that I would call again. The nurse suggested that I waited for a few minutes, as she was aware that Harry's parents were about to arrive so I sat waiting in the reception.

Tense moments

When Harry's parents arrived I stood up and reached out to shake their hands as I was introduced. I was totally unprepared for the reaction I got.

'I don't give a damn who you are,' bellowed Harry's mother. 'I haven't given you permission to come in here to see my son,' she retorted. I felt numb and not only embarrassed but also intimidated. I responded by quietly saying

'Perhaps I could have a quiet word?', to which she replied,

'I don't need a quiet word – I've told you what I think!'

I felt helpless and reasoned that if I pursued the matter further I might only aggravate what was already an unpleasant encounter. I suggested to them that I could try to explain my role. She dismissed this comment and then insisted that she spoke with my manager. Somewhat reluctantly, I gave her the team's phone number, said goodbye, and left the ward.

On reflection, the trauma experienced by Harry's parents, and his mother in particular, must have been immense. Although I had been made aware that Harry was from a close family, I had not given suffi- cient thought to the age of his parents and how they truly felt about their son's accident and his imminent move from hospital to the residen- tial home. It could, therefore, be suggested that for some parents the thought of their child seeing yet another professional when leaving home might be too much to cope with. I also thought that Harry's parents were faced with considerable conflict because not only were they trying to make the right decision for their son, but the right decision for them- selves too. They were possibly having to adjust to the impact the hospital was having on Harry and comparing it to the comforts of their home. Clearly there was a sense of responsibility on the parents' behalf to do the right thing. Their concerns, however, would determine whether their son was able to leave home and what kind of life he would lead.

Richardson (1989), Fairbrother (1986) and Richardson & Ritchie (1989), acknowledged that parents often feel that the thought of having to 'let go' of their child with a learning disability is, in fact, a great dilemma in their life and parents are so often faced with unresolved feelings of guilt, fear and uncer- tainty. Richardson & Ritchie (1989) emphasised that parents are likely to need a great deal of help during any major transition that their child goes through. It would, therefore, appear reasonable to suggest that, in order to address how parents can be supported to talk about the changes in their life, and the effect such changes may have on them, that nurses need to explore how they could offer their skills to help parents adjust rather than hinder them. I would argue that, in order to do this, certain preliminary measures must be taken into consideration with regard to the initial establishment of trust and rapport since if I am unfamiliar with the emotional experience of the parents I may hinder rather than help with the parents' adjustment.

In order to move forward in supporting Harry's parents it was necessary to reflect on my understanding of myself. Keighley (1988) suggested that it is important to understand oneself, not only as an individual but also within the context of relationships with others. Keighley also suggested that to understand and value themselves enables nurses to understand and value others.

As it happened, Harry's mother phoned my manager and complained that she was not happy that I had just turned up without an appointment at the hospital. My manager said that she explained to Harry's mother that, although she respected her concerns, she was able to see why I had made my first contact with the hospital and not with her. My manager also explained to Harry's mother the role and function of the community team. My manager informed Harry's mother that I would telephone her.

I decided that I wouldn't telephone her immediately but left it for a day. When I did phone I suggested that I met her at home where it might be easier to talk. She was calm and listened to me patiently. She asked if I would be able to visit the same day and I agreed. I was at Harry's home at least two hours, if not longer. I was made to feel welcome and was offered a drink. Harry's mother became very tearful. She expressed a great deal of remorse and repeatedly stated that she was so sorry for shouting at me in the hospital. She said that she had felt very confused. She explained that she and her husband had always done things together and that they had always involved Harry. She said she felt responsible for severing a bond that had existed for almost 40 years. She repeated herself several times as I sat quietly and listened. I simply nodded my head and offered a reassuring smile at appropriate intervals. She occasionally interjected her account by asking me to explain my role.

She asked me whether I felt that she was doing the right thing. This was such a difficult question to answer. I repeatedly asked myself how I should answer that question. Our conversation felt so intense and I felt so much responsibility. Casement (1990) suggested that intensity is the essential feature of communication in therapeutic encounters and that practitioners need to be adequately in touch with their feelings in order to work therapeutically. I would agree, in part, with this statement. However, I would also argue that it is important to retain some distance so that my impression of a situation does not become blurred.

As it happened, I dealt with the question by asking,

'What do you feel is right?'

This might seem a trite way of dealing with such an important question, but it allowed Harry's mother to reflect and prioritise what she wanted to happen. My question also helped to pursue my aim of developing trust and rapport with his mother. She responded by saying

'I want Harry to be happy and to know that we still love him.' I smiled and then said

'What do you think is right for Harry?', to which his mother replied,

'To be happy'.
'Then perhaps that is the right thing,' I added.
'You're probably right,' she said.

Time to reflect

I felt that it was important to try and get the relationship between us as comfortable as possible. This was only the first meeting with Harry's parents and I considered it to be reasonably successful. It followed what had started off as a rather unpleasant encounter but I felt that I would be able to help Harry's mother. It was a time for me to stop and question not only my practice, but also my beliefs. It was also appropriate to check out what I understood about myself.

Richardson & Ritchie (1989) commented on how the self and the environment can create unresolved stress in a situation where parents are faced with conflict of wanting to 'let go' of their child but feel restrained from doing so by overwhelming emotions of love and the fear of loss. Richardson & Ritchie and Fairbrother (1986) pointed out that the loss could often relate to the loneliness that parents experience as a result of their child moving away from home. Richardson & Ritchie, in particular, discussed how this could often hinder the ability of coping with a major life event because parents sometimes preferred their child to stay at home to fulfil their own needs of belonging and companionship. This approach may inadvertently delay the process of the parents coming to understand how to meet their own needs.

In the current situation I considered that my role was to create opportunities for Harry's parents to judge how alternative living accommodation might assist them with coming to terms with their son leaving home. Our relationship was crucial to helping Harry's parents with the changes and in determining any outcome. Leddy & Pepper (1989), and Sundeen *et al.* (1989) suggested that the emergence of any relationship between the nurse and the client can only occur once there is understanding between both parties. Therefore, outcomes cannot be determined unless there is effective communication.

The way I chose to communicate with Harry's parents was an essential component in developing trust and rapport. I felt that, in order for any trust and rapport to flourish, I needed to examine how to develop a partnership between Harry's parents, Harry and myself. Leddy & Pepper (1989) believed that this could only take place in an atmosphere of openness. Sullivan's interpersonal theory (1953) is based on the belief that human behaviour and personality develop as a result of interpersonal relationships. This theory seemed relevant to the current situation since Harry and his parents were undergoing a process of change. In these situations, relationships can foster personal growth and reduce the incidence of counterproductive behaviours.

Sullivan's theory (1953) also referred to a state of reciprocity which is concerned with a striving for satisfaction and security. Leddy & Pepper (1989) discussed this further and suggested that satisfaction occurred when biological tensions are relieved and when 'satisfaction-related' needs are met. Conversely, security is achieved when appraisals of worth, by significant others, have been acknowledged. Anxiety is also relieved when security needs are met.

The relevance of this to the current situation was that it was important that I acknowledged that I might possibly be perceived as a threat to the security and satisfaction of Harry and his parents by engineering their separation. This may have been a reason for Harry's mother's outburst on our first encounter and, had I had more time to think about this, perhaps I could have avoided any conflict. However, I was now reasonably content knowing that Harry's parents had not asked me to go when I visited them at their home. I felt that trust between us was beginning to unfold. It was important that I took hold of it so that I could work with Harry. It was also important from the point of view of determining the outcome of my intervention.

Trust is a complex phenomenon. Sundeen *et al.* (1989) stated that the concept of trust is closely related to the concept of self-awareness in that both concepts engender feelings of personal growth and discovery. When trust is experienced between two or more individuals, then all parties are able to accept one another and share information and feelings without the need to change each other. I felt that some of this was beginning to happen in my relationship with Harry's mother. Gradually, she was beginning to accept my help and support. In contrast, Richardson & Ritchie (1989) and Richardson (1989) have shown that parents often resist support in order to avoid painful thoughts and feelings.

New partners

So far, the focus of this chapter has been the relationship between Harry's parents and myself. This was necessary in order to establish trust and some clear outcomes for Harry. I have found it common in learning disability nursing that the focus of attention is someone other than the person with a learning disability. I now felt that my initial work with Harry's parents had been done and I could focus on Harry and making contact with him again.

I spent some time thinking about how I should make contact again with Harry. Amongst several important principles, the Government's White Paper, *Valuing People* (Department of Health, 2001), discussed the need for partnership working at all levels and that effective partnerships would be central to avoiding social isolation for people with learning disabilities. I would argue strongly that a partnership is an all-embracing concept that involves the acknowledgement of an individual's rights. For example, it is the individual's right not to work in partnership with professionals. Unfortunately, it is often assumed that professionals make natural partners, yet I considered it necessary to address what would make Harry want to work in partnership with me. To achieve this, I would probably need to share information about myself with Harry and try to anticipate what he might need to make the transition to his new home.

Partnership working is also a critical element of the process of empowerment. Although empowerment is perhaps an overused word, it has a great deal of resonance in the lives of people with learning disabilities, who often experience its opposite, which is a lack of control and opportunity to exercise choice (Gibson, 1991). As Gibson pointed out, it is not the role of the healthcare professional to empower other people, as only individuals can empower themselves. However, it is often the case that people need the help of others, including professionals, to feel empowered. This changes the traditional relationship between professionals and clients from one of 'power over' to one of 'power with' the client. In practice, this means careful listening on the part of the professional, giving and helping the person to understand information and securing resources, where appropriate, to improve the person's lifestyle. It is with this in mind that I arranged to meet Harry again.

I met Harry a couple of days after visiting his parents at their home. He was sitting at his bedside, flicking through some books. I greeted him and asked if I could pull up a chair to sit near him.

'Yes,' he replied.

'I'm Jackie and I'm a nurse who works outside the hospital,' I said. 'I've come to offer to help you to move from here to a new home which I understand you know about.'

'Yes,' replied Harry.

'Is that okay?' I added.

'Yes,' replied Harry.

'Are there any questions you would like to ask me?' I said.

'Are you married?' he asked.

'No I'm not,' I replied and smiled gently. I felt completely thrown.

'I've broken my leg,' he said. 'It's better now.'

I reassured Harry that it was welcoming news. At that, the trolley arrived with the afternoon tea and Harry readily accepted a drink when it was offered to him.

'Would you like a drink Jackie?' he asked.

'Thank you, that would be lovely,' I replied.

I explained to Harry that I would like to help him with his move to his new home and that it would help if he agreed to me asking him questions about himself. I told Harry that if he didn't like any of the questions I asked that he should let me know. I also told Harry that he could ask me questions to help him find out more about myself but that there might be certain questions that I would not want to answer, because I might consider them to be personal. It was agreed that we would respect each other's privacy and accept that there might be things that neither of us wished to tell each other. It was something we both regarded as important and, because it was something we had agreed, Harry put his hand out for me to shake.

I subsequently asked Harry what his feelings were about me asking other people about him and gave the example of me asking his parents. He said he didn't mind. I suggested to Harry that if I needed to ask other people questions about him that I would first discuss the matter with him so that he was aware what I would be asking and discussing with them. I also agreed to let him know of any telephone conversations or meetings with other professionals when Harry was not available. In one sense this appeared to be more important to Harry than the actual move to the home. He seemed to appreciate that a 'contract' had been negotiated between us and that he had some control over the way I supported him. In many respects it seemed that our agreement clarified the direction we needed to take and because of this it felt that we were establishing trust in one another. I was able to observe, as the weeks went by and the time for Harry to move drew closer, that there was a distinct emergence of emotional growth demonstrated by positive behavioural changes within him. This was quite a strain on his parents because suddenly their 'little boy' was speaking up for himself.

I felt it important that Harry and I should begin to get used to sharing our feelings. Keighley (1988) provided a useful exercise to help with understanding each other. The idea was that we both thought of something that had either irritated or made us angry during the past week and then pretended to be someone else in order to look at what had angered us from someone else's perspective. This appeared really beneficial for Harry. He reported that he felt that his parents were constantly suggesting what he should do. The exercise also helped Harry to appreciate more why his parents wanted certain things done for him. This in turn helped considerably with getting his point across to his parents in a non-threatening way. It also helped from the point of view of building Harry's self esteem.

Next steps

I felt that both Harry and myself now had a good foundation from which to gather information about his health needs to pass on to the care manager. Although we did not have a formal contract, we had a verbal agreement from which we could take steps to collect relevant information. We had what I felt was a sufficient knowledge of each other and an agreement of what the outcomes would look like. I also discussed with Harry that it would probably prove beneficial to evaluate our progress regarding the health profile at regular agreed intervals.

Harry and I were enjoying our meetings but they could be overshadowed by his parents' demands and his mother, in particular, wanting to know what we had discussed. I hadn't raised the importance of confidentiality with Harry's mother and father and I knew that tackling it head on would probably hinder the progress that we had all made. It was difficult at first to find a satisfactory reason to tell them why I could not share certain information with them. According to Dimond (1990), an individual is entitled to confidentiality of the information about themselves. I felt that it was necessary to explain to Harry's parents my position and to help them understand why I could not disclose information to them that Harry had shared with me. I discussed with Harry that it would appear sensible to have a small meeting with his parents where I could explain the reason why information Harry shared was confidential and that Harry could tell his parents that he did not wish them to know certain things we discussed. Harry did, however, feel that there probably would be things that he wanted his parents to know.

I arranged a meeting at Harry's parents' home and I shared with them my concerns regarding issues relating to confidentiality. It was difficult at first to know whether his parents accepted what I said but I felt I just needed to give them time to give the matter some thought. I can say, however, that they didn't disagree and they certainly did not get annoyed. I acknowledged that I needed to continue to support them in order that they could learn to accept that Harry was making very clear and definite choices about his life. It was several days later when I was in the office that I received a phone call from Harry's mother asking if I could call round to see her. She said that she had something that she wanted to discuss with me and that she couldn't talk about it over the telephone. She appeared in a state of calm and so I didn't worry that she was angered by what I had discussed the previous week. As I pulled into their drive, I noticed Harry's mum standing by the front door. I raised my hand and smiled, and parked my car. As I walked towards her she held out her arms and took hold of my right hand. She clutched it in both of her hands and repeatedly said 'thank you'.

All's well…?

I felt that I had been standing on their doorstep for at least ten minutes but in reality, it was probably only a minute. She then gave me an enormous hug.

'Come on in my dear,' she said. 'We would like you to have a cup of tea with us.'

I must admit I was really quite overwhelmed, but not to the extent that I was showing any signs of overt emotion; I was conscious that I maintained my composure at least. Harry's mother proceeded to tell me that she was so sorry for being angry with me when we first met. She said,

'I was horrible to you.'

I told her not to worry or reproach herself about it because I felt happy that we had moved on and that our move was in the right direction. I felt that the visit to their home, drinking cups of tea and eating home-made cake, was so important to Harry's parents. During the couple of hours I was with them they told me a great deal about their life together. They said that they wanted the best for Harry and that I was important to them, in helping them come to terms with all the changes.

Several weeks passed and the health needs assessment had been completed and passed on to the care manager. Afternoon visits were arranged for Harry to visit his new home and to meet his new carers. Initially, his parents joined him but as he familiarised himself with the new staff and they involved him in activities his parents gradually resisted the need to accompany him.

The day when Harry was due to leave the hospital was filled with different emotions. It had been an emotional roller coaster for many of us but Harry was happy and that was what mattered. I learnt so much from this experience that it confirmed that, regardless of how much I might know about how to support someone leaving home and, how much clinical experience I have, my work never fails to challenge me to enquire further about what I know about myself and what my perception is of others. My first encounter with Harry's parents had seemed like a disaster but my persistence and appreciation of a parent's viewpoint eventually resulted in a positive outcome for both Harry and his parents. My experience also showed the importance of establishing and maintaining a trusting relationship with both Harry and his parents. When trust exists between a professional and a client, then both parties are able to be honest and feel secure and develop as individuals.

References

Casement, P. (1990) *Further Learning from the Patient; The Analytic Space and Process.* Routledge, London.

Department of Health (2001) *Valuing People: A New Strategy for Learning Disability for the 21st Century.* Department of Health, London.

Dimond, B. (1990) *Legal Aspects of Nursing.* Prentice Hall, London.

Fairbrother, P. (1986) *Parents, Professionals and Mentally Handicapped People – Approaches to Partnership.* Croom Helm, London, Sydney.

Gibson, C.H. (1991) A concept analysis of empowerment. *Journal of Advanced Nursing,* **1**, 354–61.

Keighley, L. (1988) Self awareness. *Nursing,* **27**, 41–2.

Leddy, S. & Pepper, J. (1989) *Conceptual Bases of Professional Nursing.* J.B. Lippincott Co, London, Philadelphia.

Richardson, A. (1989) 'If you love him let him go'. In: Brechin, A. & Walmsley, J. (eds) *Making Connections.* Hodder & Stoughton, London, Sydney.

Richardson, A. & Ritchie, J. (1989) *Letting Go.* Open University Press, Milton Keynes.

Sullivan, H.S. (1953) *The interpersonal theory of psychiatry.* W.W. Norton, New York.

Sundeen, S.J., Stuart, G.W., Rankink, E.A.D. & Cohen, S.A. (1989) *Nurse–Client Interaction: Implementing the Nursing Process.* C.V. Mosby Co, St Louis, Washington, DC.

Chapter 8

A home of their own: supporting a tenants' group

Stephen Rawlinson

Introduction

I entered what was then called 'mental handicap' nurse training in 1981 at a time of momentous change with the demise of traditional hospital practice fast approaching. In its place was the challenge of an exciting new era of community-based living and caring for people who had lived for many years in an inappropriate environment. At least, that is how it seemed to myself and other students in the fledgling stage of their nursing careers. To many of the longer-serving staff the prospect of hospital closures met with much scepticism and grave misgivings, which raised questions about the efficacy of community care and the degree of risk to which vulnerable people were to be exposed. Residents, it was widely believed, were safer in hospital and, besides, society was unwilling to tolerate or accept them, and they would almost certainly be treated in a patronising, derisory or pitiful way. A core group of staff, with a vested interest in keeping the hospitals open, would not be convinced otherwise.

However, stepping into the unknown is itself a risk, without which there can be no progress or development for both individual residents and the service as a whole. Having to leave familiar surroundings and traditional working patterns, and having to undertake new roles and responsibilities was understandably stressful and threatening and required sensitive preparation and support in order to facilitate change. As a student nurse, this transitional stage seemed full of inconsistencies and contradictions. We had to abide the segregated, overcrowded and custodial conditions of hospital life whilst at the same time learn to embrace more enlightened concepts of care. In many ways, work on the hospital wards was littered with examples of bad practice, often resulting from block treatments and regimented care. Paradoxically, this has helped as reference to 'what not to do' throughout my career.

In due course, I got my chance to leave the hospital and work in a community learning disability team. In order to make care and support work outside hospital environments, nursing geared itself towards supporting families and carers of people with learning disability, who had for many years been neglected and felt overwhelmed by the problems of caring alone. Apart from a local authority day centre there had been little in the way of specialist help and support. The mainstream services that were available tended to be difficult to access due to the prevailing attitudes of the healthcare system and inability to cope with, and accommodate, those with special or challenging needs.

The move into the community was a time of confronting and challenging negative images and stereotypical ways of thinking about people with disabilities. This was necessary in order to promote community acceptance and more valued lifestyles alongside their non-handicapped peers. It was a sizeable task and one which the community team members felt somewhat ill-equipped to deal with, despite high motivation and enthusiasm. Striving to achieve comprehensive services and integration also seemed a race against time, with much ground to cover. We busily set about exploiting naturally occurring opportunities in the community and facilitated access to a variety of age-appropriate activities and experiences for people. This involved contacting and joining the local youth club, adult education classes, leisure and recreational groups, and providing employment opportunities. It was by means of sharing in the life of the local community and exposure to more natural influences that skill, competence, and relationships could develop and prosper.

The closure of hospitals, resulting mainly from adverse publicity and the discredited medicalised model meant increased pressure to develop appropriate alternatives to hospital care. In developing residential services, the general consensus was that housing for groups of six residents would be more acceptable and offer better quality care than their larger institutional counterparts. However, this small residential home model of service seemed largely a pragmatic response to an institutional problem. Though compatible groups of people were chosen, with similar needs, it was nevertheless service-driven, with little or no choice for individuals about the kind of house they lived in, the people they lived with, and how they were supported. Despite the best efforts of staff to provide active support and meaningfully engage with individual residents, evidence emerged that living in ordinary housing did not, in itself, guarantee community participation. In fact, such homes have, over the years, taken on distinctly institutional characteristics. One major drawback of residential care homes is that residents have little or no security of tenure, and often get moved for organisational reasons, or in the case of deteriorating health or behaviour.

Having a home of your own is a natural outcome of the process of change from hospital care and, for the most able clients with minimum support needs, moving into the community meant having to find suitable alternatives to the standard model of residential care. In the 1980s and 1990s this was often difficult to achieve, with perverse financial incentives in favour of residential care placements resulting in only small-scale innovation. Furthermore, despite the importance of individual planning, suitable properties were normally found prior to selecting people to fill them, with housing and support needs being inextricably bound together.

The last two decades have been characterised by unprecedented organisational change, with first the polarisation and then the vacillation between health and social care, often leaving practitioners feeling uncertain about their contribution in the field of learning disability. The overall impression is that local services are driven more by funding structures than people's needs. A mixed economy of care and the growth of the independent sector has undoubtedly created more diverse provision, but at a cost. The 'contract culture' and the tendency of purchasing authorities to buy in bulk, for instance, has stifled innovation and prevented individuals accessing the kinds of services they actually want. The shifting balance of funding away from social services to local authority housing departments, and the subsequent growth of social housing organisations, has also had a significant impact on service developments (Griffiths, 1995).

The Government is now committed to creating a society based on inclusion, independence, and empowerment (Department of Health, 1997). These principles are embodied in the recent White Paper, *Valuing People* (Department of Health, 2001), with an emphasis on developing partnerships and greater service user involvement. Though resident involvement is making great advances and is a major component of the Government's *Best Value* initiative, it is questionable to what extent learning disability nurses are actively involved in this process.

Amongst the developments in housing provision, tenant participation (TP) is now at the cutting edge of the local authorities' agendas and is valued because of its potential in making a fundamental difference to quality of life for supported housing tenants. For this client population it means new opportunities to shape and influence the quality of services they receive. It also represents a turning point in the way special needs tenants are now perceived by housing organisations as ordinary citizens with rights.

This chapter now describes the establishment of a tenants' group for people with learning disability living in supported accommodation in mid-Devon. It outlines the difficulties I encountered in formalising and helping to run the tenants' group, and establishing a framework for managing change. Identifying and addressing the problems and issues faced by special needs tenants emphasises the importance of proper consultation through listening to everyday concerns and actively supporting responsible citizenship. This seems paramount if integration policies are to take effect at a grass-roots level.

The findings of the group and the common issues raised have wider implications in terms of the way services currently operate and might change, especially as they relate to service-driven, narrowly focused individualised care approaches that mitigate against mutual support and collective action. Though positive outcomes were in evidence throughout the project, the need for extra support, training and resources, and a change in service priorities were strongly indicated.

Policy context

A major aim of the community care reforms (Department of Health, 1990) was to provide a mechanism for joint planning and collaboration, as well as better provision of information for vulnerable service users. However, despite the commitment to develop partnerships and user-centred services, their right to participate in the decision-making process has remained limited and tokenistic. The rhetoric of greater user-involvement has not only raised expectations but, in a finance-driven care system where clients have little say or status, needs are identified which clearly cannot be met. The reasons for the slow progress in redressing the balance of power between service providers and users are complex (Dowson, 1997). There is not the space here to do full justice to the various findings, but key elements clearly stand out:

- Professional protectionism and the resistance to change traditional working patterns, boundaries and power relationships (Titchen & Binnie, 1993; Sines, 1995).
- The drift towards more 'managerialism' (Thornton, 1995) and the potential for ideological conflictual relations (Malin, 1997).
- The health-social care divide creating fragmented care delivery and inflexible support (Northway, 1996).

Supporting individual rights and enhancing autonomy further requires a fundamental change in attitude, as well as acquiring skills and knowledge to operate within a new framework of care practice.

Significantly, the paucity of information and lack of central guidance for practitioners applying collaborative and user-empowerment approaches based on equal partnerships has also been highlighted (Wilson, 1993). In this context, the rapid growth of self-help, citizen and self-advocacy groups throughout the UK in the 1990s reflected a growing disillusionment with receiving the right kind of support from formal services. Few would disagree that such groups fill a gap between felt need and available services and, with a resurgence in the rights of consumers, provide an alternative platform, and indeed a theoretical framework, for gaining recognition and empowerment. Empowerment is described by Adams (1990) as:

'the process by which individuals, groups and/or communities become able to take control of their circumstances and achieve their own goals, thereby being able to work towards maximising the quality of their lives.' (p. 43)

Integral to this definition of empowerment is the concept of self-help, enablement and enhanced autonomy. It is little wonder, therefore, that with more people with learning disability living in local neighbourhoods, the challenge of empowerment has emerged as a fundamental issue in learning disability nursing (Sines, 1995). In this respect, the need to establish nurse-client partnerships seems pivotal if ambitions of achieving user-empowerment are to be realised.

Traditionally, people with learning disabilities have routinely been denied the right to a normal social life and living options have usually been restricted to residential care homes with little opportunity for extending social contacts (Simons, 1995). Furthermore, studies of hospital resettlement have found little evidence that, once living in the community, people with learning disability continue to develop new competencies and relationships, or increase participation in local affairs (Cambridge *et al.*, 1994; Emerson & Hatton, 1994; Donnelly *et al.*, 1996). Anecdotal evidence further suggests similar outcomes to those moving from the family home into ordinary housing projects (Simons, 1997). The finding that simply relocating individuals from hospital environments into community settings is unlikely to significantly affect quality of life, or ensure integration into the wider community, raises policy issues concerning the development of comprehensive community-based services. It also has practice implications for care staff in terms of role development and their ability to extend life opportunities and increase community involvement for clients in their care. With responsibility for meeting housing and social needs, service managers, too, may need to review local priorities in order to focus on individual experience and address inconsistencies in service delivery.

Carnaby Close scheme

Carnaby Close is a community-based, warden-assisted supported housing scheme for adults with learning disability and provides special needs dwellings for up to 15 people. It is small scale and a good example of what can be achieved through joint planning initiatives, involving transferred funds from health to local authority as part of the hospital resettlement programme and care in the community arrangements under Section 28A of the National Health Service Act, 1977. The scheme's main attraction is its ordinary location, being in an integrated setting adjacent to a modern housing estate, a primary school, a GP practice and the local hospital, all within easy reach of community facilities and the town centre.

During the preparation phase of the project, I became involved in working alongside the respective families and provided support and education in many key areas. The original aims of the scheme were to support more independent living and promote social integration. This philosophical approach to learning disability services embraces the idea of genuine participation of service users in the mainstream of life, recognising their right to be treated as ordinary citizens (Towell, 1988).

Living in ordinary housing provides opportunities to learn new skills, build social networks and friendships, and access mainstream resources. Though falling short of this ideal lifestyle, there have, nevertheless, been real achievements made by individual residents. The cornerstone for the scheme's progress has been the close working relationship between the warden and the community learning disability team based on a hospital site nearby of which I was a member. Certainly, the close proximity of the community team helped facilitate a rapid response to any emerging problems or crises. The team became involved in assessing people's needs and aspirations through a process of individual programme planning, and continued training in daily living skills and risk-taking have also contributed to increasing residents' independence.

However, in the context of promoting independence, fulfilling a caring role is significantly different to undertaking a role as advocate and enabler (Malin & Teasdale, 1991; Skelton, 1994). Though distinctions often blur, the former involves providing care and doing things for, whereas the latter implies doing things with, sharing power and promoting citizenship (Skelton, 1994). As Jack (1995) observed in discussing empowerment in community care, services can be a source of disempowerment by underplaying the crucial role of mainstream services in determining quality of life. This is best illustrated from a tenant's perspective where the extent of participation as tenants in the wider community and influence over basic improvements in service quality has been minimal. Though personal gains have been made, the narrow focus on personal care services, and the failure to treat clients as ordinary citizens, could account for the slow development of tenant participation.

What is tenant participation?

Tenant participation is 'the process of involving tenants in decision-making, listening to what they have to say and acting on it' (Carr-Gomm Society, 1999). This can lead to a range of benefits to both tenants and organisations as illustrated in Box 8.1.

Box 8.1   Benefits of tenant participation (adapted from Keeble, 1996; Workman, 2000; data reproduced with permission).

- Promotes tenants as active rather than passive.
- Tenants can question and challenge what is happening.
- Provides a forum for mutual support.
- Helps increase confidence, assertiveness and self-esteem.
- Provides new ideas and broader outlook to services.
- Opens the door to involvement with local communities.
- Influences the way services are planned and organised.
- Enables organisations to make better decisions.
- Provides a safeguard on standards of service.

Although tenants at Carnaby Close had been involved in decision-making, this had normally been confined to particular issues such as choosing household items and equipment rather than the full range of services they receive. Certainly, the wider range of life opportunities and service options available means that tenants increasingly need the right kind of support in making informed choices about the services they receive. However, though having assured tenancies and the same rights to consultation and information as those in general needs housing, the realisation of tenant participation for this group has received scant attention from the local council.

In the wider context, supported housing tenants, as consumers, are demanding a stronger say and to be consulted on the most basic aspects of where they live (West, 1998). A study of seven Welsh supported housing schemes, including learning disability, concluded that many tenants were left in the dark about their housing rights and that many organisations viewed tenant participation as 'a desirable but non-essential issue to be dealt with after more urgent needs are met' (Keeble, 1996). Such findings concur with the present situation at Carnaby Close, indicating that, in order to raise the profile of tenant participation and improve standards for supported housing tenants, a consideration of the wider issues was required.

Promoting tenant participation involves an organisational commitment to work in partnership with tenants, to share power and resources, and to put tenants' priorities first. With perverse incentives to protect budgets, and the relative failure to work collaboratively across service boundaries to meet tenants' needs, achieving the necessary culture change has proved problematic (Howkins, 1995; Barr, 1997). The tide of unprecedented reforms in health and local authorities in recent years has compounded the situation, fuelling concerns about delivering flexible housing and support services. At local levels, the housing-social-health care divide (Arnold & Page, 1992), and the lack of joint commissioning has led to disputes over who pays for what service and a blurring of care responsibilities. The differing operational priorities are a further barrier to achieving seamless care. This is evident in the local housing department, which, burdened with administrative change, remain inward looking and resistant to promoting tenant involvement. Traditionally, housing and support needs have tended to be compartmentalised, with housing departments discharging their responsibilities by providing the bricks and mortar (Griffiths, 1988), reflecting their general exclusion from involvement in community care planning.

Since physical presence in the community does not guarantee that people lead fulfilled lives, it was vital to the scheme's success to integrate the two elements by providing dedicated warden support and a designated community nurse for each resident. However, the introduction of care management in the area in the mid 1990s brought about a radical restructuring in care delivery and, with new bureaucratic responsibilities and diffuse accountability, the scheme's original aims suffered setbacks. For instance, a prescriptive, rationing policy enforced by social services and the tighter eligibility criteria for services meant the bulk of care services were diverted elsewhere to the most 'deserving' with complex needs. Many families thought the system of prioritising care and the tighter eligibility for services was unfair and discriminatory. Their sense of injustice may have arisen, in part, from the lack of consultation. To many, it was a sobering experience, with the realisation that need was being placed within prescribed budgets, its meaning linked more to resource allocation and public accountability rather than individual client level (Lightfoot, 1995).

Care management placed significant pressures on community nurses to maintain standards of clinical care and define role development within a broader inter-agency framework. The purchaser-provider split brought added administrative burdens on existing healthcare responsibilities, with a decreased capacity to perform core tasks as caseloads increased. Relinquishing traditional spheres of control also gave rise to uncertainties about overall responsibility of funding the warden's post at Carnaby Close, with differing operational priorities of the main agencies compromising the dedicated time to oversee the scheme's progress.

Putting things right

According to Tanner (1998), the notion of independence itself, and how professionals define it, may constrain the quality of support provided. With connotations of managing on your own with little or no support, independence all too readily fulfils the criteria as a desired outcome. Though greater self-reliance is a laudable service goal, it may not be achievable in practice if considered apart from the complex interdependencies existing between clients and their community. As Moulster and Turnbull, in Chapter 5, and Thompson and Pickering, in Chapter 9, point out, people depend on others in all aspects of life and it is the importance of understanding social situations, and the pattern of relationships in which people's needs are met, that may best guide participative and empowerment strategies (Barnes, 1997).

The correlation between how a person is perceived and treated by others and how he or she behaves in the world also underpins Wolfensberger's theory (1984), in which supporting socially-valued roles is the main strategy for enhancing personal competence and social integration. Accordingly, having low expectations of a person's social abilities and achievements can restrict learning opportunities and community participation, often leading to social exclusion and marginalisation.

By definition people with learning disability have poor communication and social interaction skills and, as such, their basic needs for autonomy and mutual support often require facilitation by others. However, responding to individualised needs alone may be counterproductive if divorced from the wider social context in which people live (Tanner, 1998). Identifying a suitable interactive model of support (Turner & Coles, 1997) is therefore crucial in attempting to promote user-empowerment. As far as supporting the residents at Carnaby Close was concerned, I set about designing a model of support that was based on cooperation and modelling of behaviour, improving self-worth and confidence, how to cope with potentially stressful situations and how to adjust goals and aspirations in the face of setbacks. I believed that many of these aspects of the model could be met by introducing tenant participation to the residents.

The origin of the tenants' group at Carnaby Close was a response to several factors. First, the setting up of a help desk by social services instead of regular social work support created gaps in care delivery and meant tenants generally had less contact with professional services. Second, gaps in service provision, particularly over the main holiday periods, warranted a reappraisal of care support needs. Third, there was growing dissatisfaction among the tenants regarding the quality of support services provided.

All tenants have daily contact with the warden but some have additional difficulties requiring extra time and support. This placed an additional burden on the warden who often struggled to meet individual calls for help in a fair and equitable way. Furthermore, the demand for personal attention has had a cumulative effect, displacing other considerations necessary to improving tenants' living conditions as a whole. In this sense, there was a growing realisation that common problems and issues faced by tenants could be best dealt with through collective action.

I helped consult each tenant about the possibility of meeting together to discuss shared concerns. I helped them to set a time and a date and, in May 1999, the first meeting of the tenants' group took place at the nearby community team office. This off-site venue was chosen because it provided adequate space, privacy and facilities. To function effectively as a group, I recommended that certain formalities were observed, such as appointing key members to serve as chairperson and secretary, and deciding the frequency of meetings. There was general agreement that adopting a structured approach, and being better organised, would more effectively address problems surrounding the running of the scheme. Working together to identify deficiencies in service provision would, it was thought, be instrumental in bringing about positive change.

Although there was some confusion about how the group would operate, everyone was prepared for me to take a lead role and to assume the position of chairperson. Since I had helped to initiate the group, I agreed to guide proceedings, though I envisaged passing on the mantle of responsibility in due course in the spirit of tenant empowerment and autonomous self-help (Adams, 1990). I later discovered that this would be easier said than done. My role as facilitator was to promote a safe and mutually supportive atmosphere for discussion, ensuring everyone had an equal say in matters arising. Due to the tenants' lack of familiarity with formal group processes, the priority was to gain their trust and confidence and to help them become more comfortable with participating in the process of change. I must admit to being apprehensive about learning my new role. Ground rules were soon established, reflecting the need to take turns and to prevent those with stronger personalities from dominating more vulnerable, less vocal members. In this sense, tolerance, listening and understanding are key features in recognising the right to hold opposing views, but also supporting the right of members to remain silent. All contributions, no matter how small, were valued.

In theory, a structured, formal approach is ideal for tackling problems collectively and making the process of decision-making and goal planning by consensus easier to achieve. However, its success in practice was found to be a complicated process involving an appreciation of the different rules of engagement within a group context. Adapting to the different demands placed on tenants and helping them to become actively engaged group members, therefore required an attitudinal and emotional adjustment.

Given comprehension difficulties, an expectation to relate in more formal ways, and the exposure to a potentially stressful environment, it was important to gradually introduce tenants, albeit experientially, to the various procedures and principles underpinning task-oriented, problem-solving approaches. It was therefore agreed to take matters slowly and to interrupt proceedings if there was something the group was not clear about. Further problems were encountered by adopting a businesslike approach in respect of conceptualising and making sense of group functioning itself. Factors governing the dynamics of group behaviour and interventions can be complex (Douglas, 1985). For instance, tenants are continuously adjusting their relationships with one another according to pervading attitudes, emotions and private agendas. One concern was that assuming a leadership role would unduly influence the group process and constrain the way the group behaved and the direction it would take. Others' concerns related to the possible influence on others by virtue of my professional status and the need to model behaviours that encouraged self-directed learning.

Although a certain amount of guidance is necessary, being too directive and 'expert' might encourage passivity and 'going along' with decisions out of a sense of self-protection (Douglas, 1985). Furthermore, some members, having poor self-image, social anxiety and lacking confidence, may feel uneasy and self-conscious about entering an equal relationship with professionals (Markwick & Sage, 1997). It was therefore important, particularly from a learning point of view, to try to emphasise my participation as an 'enabling' rather than a 'leadership' role. This meant having to be sensitive about taking control and to avoid dictating the agenda.

With this in mind, the tenants were invited, in turn, to express their immediate concerns. Interestingly, these touched on matters chiefly related to personal safety and security, namely: dealing with strangers at the door, nuisance phone calls, efficiency of on-call and alarm systems, and poor outdoor lighting. Over the course of our regular monthly meetings other matters have been raised, including getting on with neighbours, unsociable noise, receiving junk mail, unscrupulous salesmen, vandalism, and ground maintenance. Due to the scheme's close proximity to a school there have also been ongoing issues related to inappropriate parking, with concerns raised about access to emergency services.

Most of these problems are familiar. However, the susceptible nature of many tenants, who are also an ageing population, meant the amount of support needed to adequately deal with everyday life situations was much more pronounced. Identifying deficits in coping with problems was only one part of the equation. A major purpose of the group was to promote strengths and abilities and build confidence, thereby empowering tenants to speak out in order to improve quality of life. This involved the recognition that sharing time, power and information with tenants was fundamental to them making informed choices and taking more control of their lives.

After a tentative start, with tenants apprehensive about their new role and often seeking validation of their contributions, the group soon began to confront real problems in the real world. Feeling their way, and receiving positive encouragement, the group's members have already demonstrated what can be achieved through collective action. By sharing ideas and delegating responsibilities, members took positive steps in setting up a neighbourhood watch scheme, agreeing a strategy for tackling the parking problems, and improving the emergency on-call service. Since many identified problems concerned practical support for improving on-site facilities, it seemed appropriate to invite a housing officer to future meetings. This direct contact proved very useful, principally because it enabled the group to look more closely at their status as tenants and to raise issues related to tenancy rights and responsibilities.

In the past the local council have tended to pay lip-service to the needs of supported housing tenants. One key issue is the information they publish, which is often presented in non-accessible forms. Many tenants are unable to read, with some having visual and/or hearing impairments, making it important for councils to pass on information in more user-friendly ways. The use of easy words, large print, short jargon-free sentences, pictures, symbols, audiotapes and videos have already been cited as examples of how this may be achieved (Gregory, 1996; People First, 1997). One measure of progress was the initiative taken by the group's secretary to use rebus symbols alongside the minutes of meetings. To support participation, tenants need practical information about the services they receive, and again, this needs to be disseminated appropriately. Instead of reinventing the wheel, information such as *Tenant's Handbook* (First Choice, 1999) and support charters (Keeble & Forbes, 1999) are highly recommended as practical guides for people with learning disability moving into supported housing[1].

---

[1] Written in plain English and illustrated, these guides include basic information on: the rights and responsibilities of being a tenant; tenancy agreements; repairs and maintenance; health and safety; making complaints; and what to expect from support services.

Driven by the government's *Best Value* initiatives (Department of Environment, Transport and Regions, 1999a), and with an agenda to increase local democracy, housing organisations are being challenged to become more tenant-focused. This will mean conducting strategic reviews of the needs of supported housing tenants and implementing action plans designed to promote partnerships and increase tenant involvement in housing policy (Mid-Devon District Council, 2000). The introduction of tenant participation compacts[2] between councils and tenants (Department of Environment, Transport and Regions, 1999b) is, therefore, a timely opportunity for the group to have their voice heard in order to influence local policy decisions and improve service delivery.

Discussion

Though in its infancy, the tenants' group has already made tangible improvements in the running of the scheme and a fundamental difference to quality of life. Setting up a neighbourhood watch scheme has been an encouraging start, and seeing the results of their actions has helped raise the tenants' expectations of what can be achieved. However, setbacks were inevitable and the group is on a learning curve in terms of recognising the complex nature of participation and negotiating barriers to progress. Because of the risk of helping make choices tenants may wish to opt out. Several tenants have stopped attending meetings for unknown reasons, though natural anxieties, lack of confidence in groups, or a poor understanding of how they can make a difference, could explain their actions.

With additional demands being placed on tenants, resolving the issue of non-attendance, and what it means to the rest of the group, warranted a re-evaluation of the intensity, structure and dynamics of the group. This resulted in modifying the pace of change, making meetings flexible and less formal, and finding ways of continuing to include absent tenants. Recognising that levels of involvement vary according to differing abilities and support needs is, of course, fundamental to continued attendance and ensuring a user-led approach. Organising leisure outings and social events, in addition to more formal group-based activities, have also been effective in developing group identity and retaining membership.

Gathering suitable information to make informed choices over matters directly affecting their lives has proved problematic. This is symptomatic of a wider problem. People with learning disability have traditionally been marginalised and disenfranchised by professionals in the decision-making pro-

---

[2] Tenant participation compacts are local agreements between a council and its tenants on how tenants can get involved collectively in shaping decisions on housing matters affecting them (Department of Environment, Transport and Regions, 2000).

cess. Furthermore, the incongruity between perpetual client-focused approaches and the slow development of participative practice with those receiving services suggests reluctance by service agencies to fully embrace the concept of user empowerment. With clients continuing to have little control over service outcomes, this further demonstrates self-interest in perpetuating the status quo.

The time-consuming nature of tenant participation implies, in order for it to work more effectively, that extra support and resources are needed. Tenant empowerment is no quick fix, but involves a long process of building confidence, trust and relationships. Furthermore, helping tenants to speak out, make meaningful contributions and take more control over day-to-day issues is dependent on developing new skills to make it happen. To heighten the profile of tenant participation and for tenants to share in and make a fuller contribution to community life, professionals need to be proactive in shifting priorities in favour of 'needs' as defined by users. This calls for a radical approach in the style of service delivery. However, with tenant participation embracing health, social and housing need, combined with the problems of inter-agency collaboration, how far this can be achieved remains unclear.

By refocusing attention on the needs, rights and responsibilities of supported housing tenants recent *Best Value* initiatives are welcome. Rather than being treated homogeneously, such tenants have differing support needs and it will be interesting to see how policy change will translate to the lives of 'special needs' tenants. In the meantime, tenants at Carnaby Close continue to face fresh challenges. Their status as council tenants has been invigorated by voicing concerns, raising awareness of common issues affecting their lives, and acting collaboratively to improve their living conditions. However, working in isolation from other tenant participation groups may eventually lead to stagnation, signalling the need to network with similar schemes in order to share experiences and build on strengths.

It is hoped that as the group moves on, greater responsibility for the running of meetings will be transferred to the tenants themselves. This accords with a fundamental principle underpinning tenant participation whereby professionals provide discreet support and do not prescribe solutions. However, concerns about the prospect of continued dependency on professional support to direct the group, and initiate change, remain. With limited resources and the absence of an independent facilitator, finding ways to minimise this over time will be challenging. With growing pressure on community learning disability nurses to develop health practice, and without a mandate to provide social care, tenant participation as an evolving process will require a commitment by local councils to work in partnership with and actively support existing tenants' groups, whatever their needs.

References

Adams, R. (1990) *Self-Help, Social Work and Empowerment.* MacMillan Education, Basingstoke.

Arnold, P. & Page, D. (1992) *Housing and Community Care.* Joseph Rowntree Foundation (Housing Research Findings No. 58), York.

Barnes, M. (1997) Families and Empowerment. In: Ramcharan, P., Roberts, G., Grant, G. & Borland, J. (eds) *Empowerment in Everyday Life: Learning Disability.* Jessica Kingsley, London.

Barr, O. (1997) Interdisciplinary teamwork: consideration of the challenges. *British Journal of Nursing,* **6**(17), 1005–10.

Cambridge, P., Hayes, L. & Knapp, M. (1994) *Care in the Community: Five Years On.* Ashgate, Aldershot.

Carr-Gomm Society (1999) *What Is Tenant Participation? Tenant Factsheet No 2.* Carr-Gomm Society, Bristol.

Department of Environment, Transport and Regions (1999a) *Best Value in Housing Framework.* DETR, London.

Department of Environment, Transport and Regions (1999b) *National Framework for Tenant Participation Compacts.* DETR, London.

Department of Environment, Transport and Regions (2000) *Tenant participation compacts: A guide for tenants.* DETR, Wetherby.

Department of Health (1990) *The National Health Service and Community Care Act.* HMSO, London.

Department of Health (1997) *The New NHS: Modern, Dependable.* HMSO, London.

Department of Health (2001) *Valuing People: A New Strategy for Learning Disability for the 21st Century.* HMSO, London.

Department of Health and Social Security (1977) *The National Health Service Act.* HMSO, London.

Donnelly, M., McGilloway, S., Mays, N., Knapp, M., Kavanagh, S., Beecham, J. & Fenyo, A. (1996) One and Two Year Outcomes for Adults with Learning Disabilities Discharged to the Community. *British Journal of Psychiatry,* **168**, 598–606.

Douglas, T. (1985) *Groups. Understanding People Gathered Together.* Tavistock Publications, London.

Dowson, S. (1997) Empowerment within Services: A Comfortable Delusion. In: Ramcharan, P., Roberts, G., Grant, G. & Borland, J. (eds) *Empowerment in Everyday Life: Learning Disability.* Jessica Kingsley, London.

Emerson, E. & Hatton, H. (1994) *Moving Out: The Impact of Relocation from Hospital to Community on the Quality of Life for People with Learning Disabilities.* HMSO, London.

First Choice (1999) *Tenant's Handbook: Welcome to your New Home.* First Choice Housing Association, Cardiff.

Gregory, W. (1996) *The Information Manual: Making information more accessible in the light of the Disability Discrimination Act.* HMSO, London.

Griffiths, R. (1988) *Community Care: Agenda For Action.* HMSO, London.

Griffiths, S. (1995) *How Housing Benefit Can Work for Community Care: Conclusion for Policy Makers and Practitioners.* Joseph Rowntree Foundation, York.

Howkins, E. (1995) Collaborative Care: An agreed goal, but a difficult journey. In: Cain, P. & Hyde, V. (eds) *Community Nursing: Dimensions and Dilemmas,* 66–89. Arnold, London.

Jack, R. (1995) Empowerment in community care. In: Jack, R. (ed) *Empowerment in Community Care.* Chapman & Hall, London.

Keeble, M. (1996) *It Seems Like Common Sense To Me: Supported Housing Tenants Having A Say*. Tenant Participation Advisory Service (TPAS: Wales), Cardiff.

Keeble, M. & Forbes, D. (1999) *Knowing Where You Stand: Agreements for supported housing organisations and residents*. Pavilion Press, Brighton.

Lightfoot, J. (1995) Identifying needs and setting priorities: issues of theory, policy and practice. *Health & Social Care*, **3**, 105–14.

Malin, N. (1997) Policy to practice: a discussion of tension, dilemma and paradox in community care. *Journal of Learning Disabilities for Nursing, Health and Social Care*, **1**(3), 131–40.

Malin, N. & Teasdale, K. (1991) Caring versus empowerment: considerations for nursing practice. *Journal of Advanced Nursing*, **16**, 657–62.

Markwick, A. & Sage, J. (1997) Self-image and people with learning disabilities. *British Journal of Nursing*, **6**(2), 99–102.

Mid-Devon District Council (2000) *Action Plan for Tenant Participation*. MDDC, Tiverton, Devon.

Northway, R. (1996) The health and social care divide: bridging the gap. *Nursing Standard*, **10**(21), 43–7.

People First (1997) *Access first: a guide on how to give written information for people with learning difficulties*. People First, London.

Simons, K. (1995) *My Home, My Life: Innovative approaches to housing and support for people with learning difficulties*. Values into Action, London.

Simons, K. (1997) Residential Care, or Housing and Support? *British Journal of Learning Disabilities*, **25**(1), 2–6.

Sines, D. (1995) Empowering consumers: the caring challenge. *British Journal of Nursing*, **4**(8), 445–8.

Skelton, R. (1994) Nursing and empowerment: concepts and strategies. *Journal of Advanced Nursing*, **19**, 415–23.

Tanner, D. (1998) Empowerment and care management: swimming against the tide. *Health and Social Care*, **6**(6), 447–57.

Thornton, C. (1995) The changing face of management. In: Cain, P. & Hyde, V. (eds) *Community Nursing: Dimensions and Dilemmas*. Arnold, London.

Titchen, A. & Binnie, A. (1993) Changing power relationships between nurses: a case study of early changes towards patient centred nursing. *Journal of Clinical Nursing*, **2**, 219–29.

Towell, D. (1988) *An Ordinary Life in Practice*. King's Fund Centre, London.

Turner, M. & Coles, J. (1997) Meeting the needs of people with learning disabilities: developing an interactive model of care. *Journal of Learning Disabilities for Nursing, Health and Social Care*, **1**(4), 162–70.

West, T. (1998) Tenants want more say. *Housing Today*, **80** (23 April), 4.

Wilson, J. (1993) Vital yet problematic. Self-help groups and professionals: a review of the literature in the last decade. *Health and Social Care*, **1**(4), 211–18.

Wolfensberger, W. (1984) A reconceptualization of normalization as social role valorization. *Mental Retardation*, **34**(2), 22–6.

Workman, A. (2000) *Involving People with Learning Disabilities*. First Choice Housing Association Ltd, Cardiff.

Further reading

Devon Social Services Directorate (1999) *Care Management: A Differentiated Approach*. Devon Social Services, Exeter.

O'Brien, J. & Tyne, A. (1981) *The Principle of Normalisation: A foundation for effective services*. The Campaign for Mentally Handicapped People, London.

Ryan, J. & Thomas, F. (1987) *The Politics of Mental Handicap*. Free Association Press, London.

Simons, K. (2000) *Pushing open the door: Housing options: The impact of a 'housing and support' advisory service*. Joseph Rowntree Foundation, York.

Social Services Inspectorate (1991) *Care Management and Assessment: Practitioners' Guide*. HMSO, London.

Chapter 9

The relevance of learning disability nursing

Jeanette Thompson and Sharon Pickering

Introduction

The Government has established a clear agenda for all welfare services, the key elements of which centre around the need to modernise services in order to provide a quality experience for those people who use them. Central to achieving this agenda is the need to consider the following issues.

- Quality and best value
- Consumer and public involvement
- Partnership
- New ways of working
- Managing risk
- Accountability and self-regulation
- Lifelong learning

All of the above are central to the provision of quality services per se and as such are relevant to practitioners working in the area of learning disability. Although this chapter does not explore these explicitly, these areas form the central tenet of good management of service provision. In practice services are integrated with each other in order both to improve the experience of people using welfare services as well as place clients central to all that happens around them. For learning disability services the modernisation agenda is a particular challenge, mainly as a result of the diverse nature of service providers and the interface between health and social care providers.

From a nursing perspective balancing the imperatives from the sometimes parallel yet different agendas, the need to place service-users at the centre of care delivery and the political agenda can be a particular challenge that can cause significant personal conflict. Achieving this balance involves professionals in a number of the issues relating to the modernisation agenda, not least accountability and self-regulation, quality and lifelong learning.

A further issue in the move to modernise service provision is the current skill mix within services. Learning disability services have a high proportion of non-professionally qualified staff delivering direct care and support to people who have a learning disability. Whilst strategies and systems are now in place to begin to address this issue, this has been problematic on occasions (British Institute of Learning Disabilities, 2003).

Another feature of current policy is the emphasis on health issues and people with learning disabilities. Historically, learning disability nursing has always been focused upon meeting a range of needs of people who have a learning disability. Implicit within this was the belief that the health needs of this group of people were included and were being adequately met. This is of significant importance as it is now understood that this group of people have greater health needs than the rest of the population (Department of Health, 2001a). Reflecting upon past trends in learning disability services and upon learning disability nursing in particular does, however, suggest that in some instances this has not been addressed as well as it might nor has it necessarily been dealt with in the same way as is the case for the rest of the population (Turner & Moss, 1995; Lindsay, 1998).

As a consequence of recent research into the health needs of people who have a learning disability there has been an increased focus on the health needs of this population. Ultimately this has resulted in the inclusion of health within the White Paper *Valuing People: A New Strategy for Learning Disability for the 21st Century* (Department of Health, 2001a). Within this document four key principles are identified. These are:

- Choice
- Independence
- Rights
- Inclusion

Valuing People makes a clear statement that each of these principles should underpin every aspect of service delivery and all developments within the area of learning disabilities. Nowhere is this more important than in meeting the health needs of the learning disability population. Key within *Valuing People* is the intention to mainstream the way in which the health needs of this group of people are met. This crucial agenda is not only influenced by the *Valuing People* White Paper but also by a multitude of other political imperatives. Most important of these are the drives to modernise the healthcare system in its broadest sense. Within this, the public involvement and the patient liaison and advice services are fundamental. More generic policy directives, such as inclusion, also add weight to this process.

It is the intention of this chapter to explore many of these directives in the context of learning disability nursing, as well as consider the fundamental principles outlined within the Government's White Paper *Valuing People*. This discussion will, wherever possible, be supported by material drawn from other chapters within this text that explore both the journey, the values and the skills of a number of practitioners in the field of learning disabilities.

Underlying principles

Inclusion

Towards the end of the last century the Government acknowledged the level of social exclusion that existed within the United Kingdom compared to other European countries. Within other chapters in this book there are numerous examples that demonstrate ways in which people who have a learning disability have experienced social exclusion. Particularly good examples of this include Judith who, in Chapter 6, is introduced by Peter Dawson as a woman who very clearly knew that she wanted to live in her own place and, for much of her life, was prevented from achieving this by the structures and systems that surrounded her. Whilst Judith eventually got what she wanted, what is important today is that we question how many other people are still living in similar circumstances. Situations where people are clearly isolated from the rest of society simply because the systems and structures around them deem that they could not or should not be part of society, are clearly not inclusive. It would be quite reassuring to feel that this was a one-off but many of the other chapters indicate that people have had experiences that have also meant that they have been excluded in some way or another from different aspects of society.

Social exclusion can occur for a variety of reasons. As Jill Turner points out in Chapter 3, Sue limited herself and her social opportunities as a result of her continence issues. This aptly demonstrates the importance of support for people who have a learning disability to meet their health needs. It is for reasons such as this that health was seen as such a central part of *Valuing People*. Within the White Paper there was an acknowledgement that without good health people could not enjoy many aspects of life that others have long recognised to be important. This was also reinforced by Anya Souza (Souza, 2001) when she talked about the need to be healthy to be happy and, conversely, the need to be happy to give 'us' a reason to be healthy. Social inclusion is part of what she described as the reason to be healthy: in other words, having friends.

Particular aspects of exclusion that the Government has acknowledged include poverty and low income, both of which are pertinent for many people who have a learning disability. As a result of the acceptance that such issues influenced a person's ability to become involved within their society the

Government established a social exclusion unit. This unit has defined social exclusion as:

> '. . . a shorthand term for what can happen when people or areas suffer from a combination of linked problems such as unemployment, poor skills, low incomes, poor housing, high crime, bad health and family breakdown'.
>
> (For more information, see their website, www.socialexclusionunit.gov.uk)

The Government has accepted that this is a particularly flexible definition and perceived it as useful, especially as many of the factors influencing social exclusion can be mutually reinforcing. In creating this, mutual reinforcement situations can become complex and quickly result in the creation of a vicious circle or self-fulfilling prophecy. In order to try to address this situation the social exclusion unit established three key goals, which are:

(1)   Preventing social exclusion happening in the first place by reducing risk factors and acting with those who are already at risk.
(2)   Reintegrating those who become excluded back into society.
(3)   Delivering basic minimum standards to everyone, in health, education, work, income, employment, and tackling crime.

When working to meet each or all of these agendas new ways of working are often initiated in order to create some of the more creative approaches to the issue of social inclusion. The changing workforce programme aims to have a consistent and rigorous approach to modernising the workforce across both health and social care (www.doh.gov.uk/chpo/workforce.htm).

Preventing social exclusion

None of the chapters in this book provide us with clear examples of preventing social exclusion. However, some of the chapters do give us clear examples of people striving to support people to be more involved with the society in which they live. One of the good examples of this is included within Rebecca Welsh's account in Chapter 12, where she describes the importance of personal achievement in stimulating confidence and determination. This particular example focuses upon a young woman who attended an activity centre where she was supported to go down a man-made pothole. Whilst for most people this experience took 15 minutes, for this lady, who had cerebral palsy, it took three hours. The sense of achievement she felt is reported to have prompted her to move on, by going to college and moving into her own home, where she employed her own supporters. This woman now appears to have a lifestyle that would prevent social exclusion and would give her a good quality of life. Within the context of achieving a modernised welfare service it is apparent within this example that management of risk was a clear issue for this woman and that lifelong learning was stimulated for both the woman and for Rebecca. What is also important within this example is that the initial empowering act occurred within what would now be termed 'natural support systems', which are places that most of us use and gain value from.

Reintegrating people back into society

An excellent example of reintegrating people back into society is provided by Peter Dawson in Chapter 6, where he and his team worked very hard to listen to Judith and to help her to achieve her goal of moving into her own home. Peter's account showed how it could be difficult to continue to listen to Judith and work within the system where there are individuals who are determined to prevent people like her from achieving their goal. If what Peter and his team did were to be translated into today's language and belief systems, they would be seen to be operating in a person-centred way and to be empowering the person to strive to achieve what they wanted in life. This example really demonstrates the value and importance of individuals within systems: not just Judith but also the professionals working within systems. Examples such as this show that each individual has the power to influence change, whatever their role. The important factor is for them to live up to their beliefs and values, to listen to people who have a learning disability and not to give up in the face of conflict and adversity.

In Chapter 2, Tim Riding refers to working with Alan, who has a history of offending, and he describes the process that they engaged with in order to ensure that Alan was able to return to the community. In addition, Colin Doyle's goal in working with Megan (see Chapter 4) was to help her to achieve a behaviour pattern that would be seen as socially acceptable in order to support her inclusion in her community. From both these examples it is possible to see how lifelong learning is important for both the service users and the practitioners working with them.

In Chapter 11, Adrian Jones describes a different approach to reintegrating people back into society. In his chapter he focuses upon how mainstream NHS services meet the needs of people who have a learning disability. Whilst it is apparent in the first instance that this was not a wholly positive experience for Julie, the optimistic message is the willingness of the services involved to learn from their mistakes and to implement change to try and ensure this situation would not be repeated.

Delivering equitable services

Again, Adrian Jones' chapter looks at how a person who has a learning disability might receive the same services as the rest of society within acute health services. There are also a number of other examples within the chapters which describe how learning disability nurses strive hard to ensure that the people they are supporting have equity of access, particularly to welfare services. In particular, in Chapter 3 Jill Turner ensures that she regularly supports Sue to visit her general practitioner and have all the appropriate tests in order to arrive at an appropriate diagnosis. Rebecca Welsh, in Chapter 12, demonstrates the vital role she plays in supporting Tristan to access neurological services in his local hospital. Implicit within these examples are issues relating to lifelong learning, accountability and self-regulation within nursing. This is particularly relevant, for example, as Jill acknowledges within her chapter the level to which her knowledge base increases regarding continence issues as a result of her work with Sue. Likewise, Julie Wilkins, in Chapter 10, acknowledges how much her knowledge of sexual health and women's issues increased through her work with Jenna. Although these examples focus on how nurses ensure the people that they support receive equitable health services, there are many instances when learning disability nurses support people they work with to access a whole range of other services including education and valued employment.

Social exclusion and valuing people

The White Paper *Valuing People* picks up on the issues of social exclusion facing people who have a learning disability and it notes the following issues:

- *Health needs:* people who have a learning disability have greater health needs while at the same time visit their GP less frequently and have variable experiences with mainstream healthcare services.
- *Housing:* this is identified as a key issue in achieving social inclusion. For people who have a learning disability the number who are supported to live independently in the community is small. Many are given no real choice and very little information about housing options.
- *Day services:* many day services offer very limited services often equating to warehousing or containment. Services are only rarely provided on a flexible and person-centred way.
- *Social isolation:* this remains a perennial problem for people who have a learning disability, with one study identifying that only 30% had a friend who was not disabled, not a family member nor paid to care for them (Emerson *et al.*, 1999).
- *Employment:* this is an area many of us rely upon to provide the means to live the rest of our lives in the way we choose. For people who have a learning disability only 10% are in any sort of employment, this results in an unemployment rate of 90% – significantly higher than any other part of society. Employment or lack of employment not only has a significant impact on a person's level of social inclusion but also on their overall health and wellbeing (Thompson & Pickering, 2001).

Other factors affecting social exclusion addressed by *Valuing People* include the needs of people from minority ethnic communities, families with disabled children, young disabled people at the point of transition to adult life and carers.

Within *Valuing People* and the associated healthcare agenda, inclusion is a key principle, which influences the strategic direction in which services should be developing. As already discussed, this document and the subsequent guidance that was published (Department of Health, 2001b) gives a clear message that people who have a learning disability should be able to have their health needs met in the same way as any other member of the general population. This has clear implications for both specialist learning disability services as well as mainstream NHS services. Learning disability services need to be considering the ways in which they can now support their colleagues in other services to meet the health needs of this group of people. In addition, mainstream NHS services need to contemplate how their services, practices and attitudes to people who have a learning disability can and will influence the quality of service delivered.

Choice and control

Choice is a principle that has long held resonance within learning disability services; it was fundamental to Wolfensberger's principles of normalisation and social role valorisation (Wolfensberger, 1972). It also formed a crucial tenet in the works of John O'Brien. In his work O'Brien (1987) stated that choice is the experience of growing autonomy from both everyday decisions through to the larger more life defining events. It could be argued that personal choice defines an individual's total being. Therefore, the concept of choice is vital with regard to the provision of services and the roles of learning disability nurses.

More recently choice has been presented as a central plank of person-centred planning in the White Paper, *Valuing People* (Department of Health, 2001a). Within *Valuing People* choice is noted as one of the four key principles upon which all services and individual practitioners' interventions should be built. Further to this the Government's objective within this document was to enable people who have a learning disability to have as much choice and control over their lives as possible. This includes the person being able to exercise choice and control over the services and the support they have. Clearly this is demonstrated with significant success in Peter Dawson's chapter where the whole focus of the work with Judith was to listen to her and to empower her to take control over her own life. Similarly, Stephen Rawlinson, in Chapter 8, spent time listening to the tenants' group to discover what they wanted and needed to help them function as a group. Examples such as this focus very clearly upon service-user involvement in the development of services from an individual perspective. As such, therefore, this can be seen to interface with the broader Government agenda of consumer and public involvement.

Despite the length of time that people have been advocating choice as the essence of good practice within learning disability services it could be argued that it is still something that often eludes both people who have a learning disability and those that provide services. This could be as a result of the high number of practitioners involved in supporting people who have a learning disability as this can result in the loss of autonomy and independence. This is often as a consequence of the belief that the professional or paid staff member knows best (Williams, 1993). This may also be influenced by the perception of this group of people that the person is dependent, a subject discussed in more detail later in this chapter.

The dichotomy identified here can be seen within the discourse in Peter Dawson's chapter where essentially there were two teams in conflict with one another and Judith in the middle. The difficult element within all this was that both teams professed to be acting in Judith's best interests and also to know her best. Whilst this example was set in a hospital, it is possible to imagine other situations where this could also be the case, particularly with people who have no verbal communication. The only way that these complex situations can be prevented would be first to listen to what the person is saying and, where this is difficult, ensure circles of trust are developed around people. In such circumstances it would be difficult for people such as the psychologist described in Peter Dawson's chapter to undermine the wishes of the person who has a learning disability on the basis of professional beliefs and wisdom or an unwillingness to take risks. This example identifies how difficult it may be for professionals both to take risks and manage the consequences that may ensue from these decisions.

Despite many examples of good practice, *Valuing People* has identified that people who have a learning disability have little control over their life, few receive direct payments, advocacy services are underdeveloped and people who have a learning disability are often not central to the planning process. As such, whilst many years have been spent articulating the need to offer people real choices and the opportunity to take more control over their lives and believing to a great extent that this is being achieved, there is now a need to explore just how real these choices are and how these compare with the choices available to the rest of the population. This is particularly pertinent when considered in the context of statistics such as those that demonstrate only 6% of people who have a learning disability have control over who they live with and only 15% have a choice or control over who provides the care they receive (Emerson *et al.*, 1999).

When working with Alan, Tim was aiming to return him to his local community in his own self-contained flat in a complex consisting of six flats. Within this setting the building was owned by a housing trust and the support contract was with an independent sector agency. To all intents and purposes this suggests Alan was being given an opportunity to have more choice and control over his life. However, it was not clear how much control he would have over who provided him with support. Despite this, Tim was embarking upon a complex and potentially risky plan of action in working with Alan to move him from life in a young offender institution to one within his own local community. In doing this many attempts were made to balance person-centred approaches which aimed to increase Alan's choice and control, with ensuring the safety of both Alan and the general public. This demonstrates the complexity of choice and control for some groups of people in receipt of welfare services.

At the same time as noting the difficulties Tim Riding's chapter also demonstrates the potential to succeed and what this can mean for an individual. It could be suggested that the success of this initiative is in no small part due to the willingness of the team involved with Alan to balance the legal requirements placed upon them by Alan's detention under The Mental Health Act (HMSO, 1983) and person-centred approaches to his support. Inherent within the situation described by Tim Riding are the concepts of risk management and lifelong learning and the way in which both of these concepts contribute to the wider modernisation agenda.

Person-centred approaches and person-centred planning

One of the major initiatives identified within the White Paper designed to support the increase of choice of people who have a learning disability or control over their own lives is person-centred planning (PCP) and person-centred approaches (PCAs). PCP is defined as:

'... a process for continual listening and learning, focused on what is important to someone now and for the future, and acting upon this in alliance with family and friends.' (Department of Health, 2001a, p. 2)

Whilst PCAs are defined as:

'... ways of commissioning, providing and organising services rooted in listening to what people want, to help them live in their communities as they choose.' (Department of Health, 2001a, p. 4)

From these definitions it is apparent that a subtle difference and a clear inter-relationship exists between PCP and PCAs. Whilst PCP is a process for listening and acting upon what is important for the person, PCAs are about taking that information and using it to inform the design and delivery of services.

Person-centred planning and person-centred approaches can therefore facilitate developments in the following areas:

- Helping people to say what they want to happen in their lives and build their confidence in asking for this and making it happen.
- Clarifying the support needed to make the person's wishes become reality.
- Developing partnerships between people who are involved in supporting people who have a learning disability in order to develop joint problem solving.
- Creating energy and motivation within supporters based upon hearing what the person really wants to happen in their life.
- Providing the basis from which all services should be developing.

A number of chapters describe examples of where learning disability nurses have been involved in helping the people they are working with to say what they want in their lives. The role of advocacy in this is clearly articulated within Peter Dawson's chapter, as is the importance of listening to an individual in order that the message given is one that truly reflects the wants and expectations of the person who has a learning disability.

In Chapter 7, Jackie Roberts describes a situation where a parent is uncomfortable with Jackie speaking to her son (who is 40 years old) without his mum being present. This situation highlights some of the complexities that surround this particular aspect of the role of the learning disability nurse. The balance between listening to the person at the same time as supporting their parents, who may have previously been encouraged either to place their child in an institution or to manage in difficult circumstances without much support, can be challenging. In her chapter Jackie Roberts manages to strike a careful balance with the support of her manager, in which she listens to and supports Harry's mother in order to gain a working relationship that then allows her to listen to what Harry wants to happen in his life.

Stephen Rawlinson, in Chapter 8, also shows how he helped a group of ex-hospital residents to achieve the lifestyles that they wanted outside the institution. This chapter is particularly helpful in demonstrating just how much help and encouragement people need to speak up and to begin to take control over their lives.

Clarifying support needed to make wishes a reality

Identifying the support needed by people who have a learning disability in a way that helps them to achieve what they want in life is crucial to the work of any professional. It is particularly important to ensure that support is sufficient to make sure that the person does not feel isolated or place themselves in undue positions of risk. Equally, it is important to ensure that people are not over supported and control is taken away from the person as a direct consequence of this. In Tim Riding's chapter, in which he describes the complexities of working with Alan, he is constantly having to deal with this very issue. At the time Alan meets Tim Riding he is sectioned under the

Mental Health Act, which places huge constraints upon Alan and the choices and control he is able to have over his own life. Alan is sectioned because, at the time of his detention, he was perceived as a risk to society. In order for him to return to that society in a successful and safe way it is important that appropriate support is made available to him. One of the important aspects demonstrated within this chapter is the way in which these supports may have to operate within certain parameters which may appear to deny the person some degree of choice. As with the majority of the population, Alan has to make choices based around the reality of the world that he lives in. For the professionals working with Alan, risk management is a significant part of the process underpinning the achievement of a more normative approach to life and for services it involves a more creative use of their resources in support of the inclusion agenda.

Developing partnerships

One of the key aspects of the modernisation agenda is that of partnerships. Partnerships are crucial in bringing about a seamless service that delivers what the service user wants. In all the chapters there are good examples of the development of a broad range of partnerships. Within the chapters there are partnerships between the nurse and the people they support, the nurse and other supporters, including family, friends and significant others, between teams and across agencies. Rebecca Welsh, in Chapter 12, demonstrates a range of partnerships that are crucial to meeting Tristan's needs around his epilepsy. Significant within this is the relationship Rebecca developed with Tristan's mother. In particular, it focuses upon the link Rebecca perceived to exist between his mother's reluctance to take key decisions with Tristan regarding dealing with his epilepsy and medication changes as well as any unresolved grief she may have had about the birth of a child with a learning disability. Having identified this, Rebecca spent a significant amount of her time working with Tristan's mother in order to ensure the success of any changes proposed by the neurologist. Equally both Colin Doyle, in Chapter 4, and Jackie Roberts, in Chapter 7, talk of developing key partnerships with parents and ensuring their involvement in the assessment process.

Jackie Roberts talks at length about how she established a relationship with Harry. Importantly, she notes the right of Harry not to work with her and that professionals do not always make the natural partners we would like to believe they are. Important in her considerations of how she would develop an effective relationship with Harry were her thoughts around the level of self-disclosure she would need to make to ensure a reciprocal relationship was able to develop, an essential element of valued and effective relationships that are person centred.

Creating energy and motivation

The belief within person-centred approaches to services is that the successes achieved will generate a level of energy and motivation that spurs service providers and others on to work harder and do more. In some instances this is apparent in the opening pages of each chapter as the authors describe the successful and person-centred involvement that they have had with someone who has a learning disability. Each person having had that initial experience is driven to find a way to do more and to help people achieve more for themselves. In addition, all the people who have written chapters in this book have embarked upon a process of lifelong learning. Nowhere is this more clearly articulated than in Chapter 4, where Colin Doyle frequently refers to the factors influencing further developments in his chosen career and the need to increase both his knowledge and skill base.

Underpinning for service delivery

There is a fundamental belief within services that services and supports should be developed according to what the people in receipt of that service want and need. This is apparent in a number of the chapters, notably Peter Dawson's chapter and that of Tim Riding. In both of these chapters the authors, in different ways, are trying to find out what the person wants and then use that to form the basis of the services they receive in the future. When considering the essence of consumer involvement in modernised welfare services this is part of what people are all aiming for. It is therefore reassuring to see examples of where this occurs within learning disability nursing. *Valuing People* does, however, caution us against complacency with regard to believing that we all achieve this all of the time.

In addition to person-centred planning as a way of increasing the choice and control of people who have a learning disability, the White Paper also introduced the concept of health action planning (HAP). Health action planning is to be person centred in the same way as person-centred planning. A person should have only one plan; it should be their plan, not that of the professionals. As such it should, therefore, include issues felt to be important by the person in relation to their health and should also be in a format that is understandable and accessible to them. Each of these principles should increase the choice and control the person has in relation to their life, and in turn this can be seen to be contributing to the broad expectations encapsulated within the modernisation agenda.

Independence

Promoting independence is key to the achievement of the Government's modernisation agenda as well as sitting comfortably with many of the principles and philosophies that underpin services for people who have a learning disability. Whilst it is readily acknowledged that people who have a learning disability have a wide variety of needs, and some people will continue to need significant amounts of support, it is important that the start point for work with any individual is that of independence not dependence. Independence, in this context, does not mean doing everything unsupported. In fact, interdependence may be a better description of what we are talking about in this instance.

Jefferson & Hall (1998) discuss the concept of the dependence-independence continuum. Within this they discuss the common belief that dependence and independence are mutually exclusive; a person can only be one or the other. By striving within services to promote independence as a desired goal we attach negative connotation to the idea of dependence and, as such, dependency is seen as a deviation from society's desired norm. For people who have a learning disability this societal norm has significant implications for their ability to achieve in many areas. Key aspects of this include their ability to own their own home, have a job and other things that the rest of society take for granted.

An alternative view on this is that no person is truly independent, each of us relies on someone in order to live the life we want, to the level of success we choose. For all of us a state of interdependence is inevitable and desirable. Fundamental to this concept is an acceptance that others will provide the services that some are unable to or choose for themselves. This can include things that are as much an accepted part of how society operates as 'going to the supermarket'. Such acceptance of certain aspects of support indicates the social construction that is inherent within the dependence-independence continuum. As Johnson (1990) stated, the essence of interdependence lies in the notion that everyone is reliant on others for some aspect of their daily living whether it be practically or emotionally. In addition Johnson (1990) noted that interdependence fosters cooperation, collaboration and effective teamwork. Within learning disabilities this is important, as the essence of cooperation, collaboration and effective teamwork has now been extended to include people who have a learning disability and their parents' families and friends. Changing the balance of power in this way can only be achieved if we truly embrace the concept of interdependence but with the underlying start point that dependence should not be the norm for people who have a learning disability.

There are numerous examples within the chapters of the practitioners working towards the goal of independence for the people that they are working with. However, in reality many of the examples are ones in which the concept of interdependence is implicit. In fact the greatest successes in terms of positive outcomes for the person in receipt of services are where there is a significant element of interdependence in the outcome. This is particularly evident in Peter Dawson's chapter, where it can be seen that Judith has moved from a forced dependence within the hospital setting to interdependence with both the housing association and the local church. Important within this is Judith's relationship with her male friend.

The need to change the balance of power not only between practitioners and the people that they are working with, but also between parents and children is also evident. This is particularly relevant in the situation where the parent may well feel the need to maintain their child's dependence in order to protect them. Jackie Roberts, in her chapter, acknowledges the need to work on this area with Harry's mother. So, too, does Colin Doyle in Chapter 4.

Whilst the influence of the dependence-independence continuum can and will have its impact within learning disability services the risks within mainstream services could be even greater, particularly as independence is regularly presented as the goal of nursing care. By virtue of this the risk is that people who present as not being able to do for themselves as a result of having a learning disability will be ascribed all the roles that are associated with dependence. This may also include concepts such as being asexual, unassertive and devalued. Essentially this is the premise which underpins the concept of a self-fulfilling prophecy or a vicious circle in which low expectations lead to lower achievement that, in turn, reinforces low expectations.

Making a difference to this situation is in part what the concept of health facilitation is designed to achieve. This particularly focuses upon the level of work aimed at service development and informing commissioning and planning. In doing this it is intended to support people who have a learning disability to get what they want and need from the NHS, as well as other services, that may help them to stay healthy.

Despite the fact that the concept of health facilitation is a relatively new one we can see examples of this role in an embryonic state in some of the chapters. Particularly notable is the work of Rebecca Welsh with Tristan and the neurology services, Jill Turner and Sue with the GP, and Adrian Jones from within an acute hospital trust. Whilst most of these interventions have been built around work with individuals the knock-on impact upon services for other people who have a learning disability should be evident, as is the relevance of this to partnership working.

Rights

As with choice, rights has also been one of those areas in which we have long advocated the importance of people who have a learning disability having and exerting their rights. Again, it has been discussed throughout the last 30 years of service delivery, beginning with Wolfensberger and culminating with the White Paper *Valuing People*. This document supports the Government's wider commitment to enforceable civil and legal rights for people who have a disability and identifies the relevance of this for people who have a learning disability. Also of crucial importance with regards to the rights of people who have a learning disability are a vast range of legislative bills, that include:

- The Human Rights Act (1998)
- The Disability Discrimination Act (1995)
- The Race Relations Act (1976)
- The Race Relations (Amendment) Act (2000)
- The Sex Discrimination Act (1975)
- The UN Convention on the Rights of the Child (adopted in the UK in 1992)

Fundamental to the exercise of a person's rights is the concept of citizenship. The term 'citizenship' is used to describe the establishment of statutory conditions whereby all members of society can take a full and productive role in the nation's life. Marshall (1951) described citizenship as an achievement of civil, political and social rights, as can be seen from Box 9.1.

Box 9.1   Civil, political and social rights (from Jefferson & Hall, 1998).

Civil rights
- Legal rights
- Right to contract
- Property rights
- Freedom of thought
- Freedom of speech
- Choice in religious practice

Political rights
- Universal suffrage (right to vote)
- To organise politically

Social rights
- Access to welfare services and benefits
- Standards of living in line with current social expectations

---

Within most of the chapters in this book there is evidence of the ways in which learning disability nurses are supporting people to achieve their social rights more effectively. This particularly focuses upon access to welfare services. In addition there are some examples of people being supported to achieve civil rights. This is particularly evident in Peter Dawson's chapter in which he supports Judith to speak up for herself and in which she ultimately exercises her right to choose her religion and the way in which she will practice this. It is also apparent in Tim Riding's chapter about Alan's right to contract by virtue of his tenancy agreement with the housing association and in Stephen Rawlinson's work with the tenants' group to get them to exercise their rights as tenants.

The area in which there is limited evidence of involvement by learning disability nurses is that of political rights. This does not mean that learning disability nurses are not actively involved in supporting people in this area, as can be seen from Peter Dawson's current role in supporting self advocacy (Dawson, 2002). As services develop that support people who have a learning disability to advocate for or assert themselves it is hoped that more and more people who have a learning disability could become politically active if that was their wish.

Conclusion

This chapter has explored key themes identified within the Government strategy, *Valuing People* (Department of Health, 2001a). In addition there has been discussion about where inclusion fits in with the broader Government objective relating to social exclusion and ways in which people who have a learning disability can be excluded from the society in which they live. The discussion has also explored ways in which learning disability nurses both now and in the past have contributed to the inclusion of people who have a learning disability. Further to this, the chapter has taken the concept of choice and the inter-relationship that this has with control over a person's own life and have also looked at the ways in which person-centred planning and person-centred approaches contribute to the achievement of this goal.

In relation to independence, the issue of the dependence-independence continuum has been highlighted, in particular the impact it has upon both the societal perceptions of people who have a learning disability, as well as on the way in which professionals work. In doing this, the discussion has identified the importance of the concept of inter-dependence and how this creates a much more natural goal for all members of society.

This chapter has also considered the issue of rights from the perspective of people who have a learning disability. This concept has been clearly framed within the vast legislative framework of the United Kingdom and Europe that underpins this area of work. As such, the examples from other chapters show the ease with which learning disability nurses support people in the attainment of both their social and civil rights.

Finally, this chapter has demonstrated the absolute importance of people, not just those in receipt of services, but also the importance of the values, attitudes and beliefs of those delivering services. It is only where these two groups are working in synchronicity that true achievement occurs. If this does not underline the crucial importance of people and their personalities and the impact they can have upon someone's life then what does?

References

British Institute of Learning Disabilities (2003) *The Learning Disability Awards Framework*. BILD, Kidderminster.

Dawson, P. (2002) Hearing but not listening. *Learning Disability Practice* **5** (7), 26.

Department of Health (2001a) *Valuing People: A New Strategy for Learning Disability for the 20th Century*. Department of Health, London.

Department of Health (2001b) *Valuing People: A New Strategy for Learning Disability for the 20th Century – Implementation*. HSC 2001/016: LAC (2001) 23. Department of Health, London.

Emerson, E., Robertson, J., Gregory, N., Hatton, C., Kessissoglou, S., Hallam, A., Knapp, M., Järbrink, K. & Netten, A. (1999) *Quality and Costs of Residential Supports for People with Learning Disabilities: A Comparative Analysis of Quality and Costs in Village Communities, Residential Campuses and Dispersed Housing Schemes*. Hester Adrian Research Centre, Manchester.

HMSO (1975) *The Sex Discrimination Act*. HMSO, London.

HMSO (1976) *The Race Relations Act*. HMSO, London.

HMSO (1983) *The Mental Health Act*. HMSO, London.

HMSO (1995) *The Disability Discrimination Act*. HMSO, London.

HMSO (1998) *The Human Rights Act*. HMSO, London.

HMSO (2000) *The Race Relations (Amendment) Act*. The Stationery Office, London.

Jefferson, J. & Hall, M. (1998) Promoting choice, autonomy and independence for older people. In: Pickering, S. & Thompson, J. (eds) *Promoting Positive Practice in Nursing Older People*. Ballière Tindall, London.

Johnson, M. (1990) Dependency and interdependency. In: Bond, J. & Coleman, P. (eds) *Ageing and Society*. Sage, London.

Lindsay, M. (1998) *Signposts for Success*. Department of Health, London.

Marshall, T.H. (1951) *Citizenship and Social Class*. Cambridge University Press, Cambridge.

O'Brien, J. (1987) A guide to lifestyle planning: using the activities catalogue to integrate services and natural support systems. In: Wilcox, B.W. & Bellamy, G.T. (eds) *The Activities Catalogue: An Alternative Curriculum for Youths and Adults with Severe Disabilities*. P.H. Brookes, Baltimore.

Souza, A. (2001) Being well: my well-being. In: Thompson, J. & Pickering, S. (eds) *Meeting the Health Needs of People who have a Learning Disability*. Ballière Tindall, London.

The United Nations (1992) *The United Nations Convention on the Rights of the Child*. United Nations, New York.

Thompson, J. & Pickering, S. (2001) *Meeting the Health Needs of People who have a Learning Disability*. Ballière Tindall, London.

Turner, S. & Moss, S. (1995) *The Health Needs of People with a Learning Disability*. Hester Adrian Research Centre, Manchester.

Williams, I. (1993) What is a profession? Experience versus practice. In: Walmsley, J., Reynolds, J., Shakespeare, P. & Woolfe, R. (eds) *Health, Welfare and Practice: Reflecting on Roles and Relationships*. Open University Press, Milton Keynes.

Wolfensberger, W. (1972) *The Principle of Normalisation in Human Services*. National Institute of Mental Retardation, Toronto.

Chapter 10

Taking a step back: tackling women's health issues in learning disability

Julie Wilkins

A harsh beginning

I began my career as a newly qualified staff nurse in 1984 on a 30-bed female forensic ward. I can remember being immensely proud of my uniform and shiny silver buckle, which was compulsory then, and worn to ensure that the staff were clearly distinguishable from the patients. When I look back to my early days as a young, impressionable staff nurse I reel in horror at the things I took for granted and never questioned and how quickly I became involved in the institutional regime.

I distinctly remember the drug trolley being wheeled out of the treatment room and the majority of women queuing up to receive the contraceptive pill, which was handed out like smarties without any consideration for the individual concerned. I cannot remember asking any of the women if they were sexually active, if they would like a choice of contraception, whether they would like their partner to use condoms or receive sex education. The assumption was that if women were not sexually active when they were admitted, the majority would be when the time came to be discharged. As for sex education, I guess it was presumed that most women had some knowledge that they had acquired elsewhere. In reality, most of the women had their first sexual experience with their peers soon after they were admitted. Would-be male suitors from the adjoining ward would compete for the attention of any new woman. This resulted in brief relationships and, again, no formal sex education was offered.

Relationships were quite often abusive and the women occasionally received nasty injuries on their body, including their genitalia, that often went unnoticed by the staff. On one occasion, I remember helping a 20-year-old woman to wash and style her hair. As she stood up I noticed that both her breasts were completely black where she had been punched during sexual intercourse. I think the most distressing thing of all was that she did not realise it was wrong to be punched during sexual intercourse and thought it was all part of a sexual relationship.

Many women received payments for sex, usually in the form of sweets, soft drinks and cigarettes and it was often apparent who had been providing sexual favours on pay days by the amount of 'goodies' they brought back to the ward. Women admitted to the forensic wards were aged from 18 to 60 years but the one experience that most of them had in common was that the majority of them came from homes where loving, nurturing relationships were uncommon and where many families were devoid of expressing feelings and emotions. It was hardly surprising that most women felt little enjoyment in their sexual experiences, because their expectations were low and they had nothing to compare them to. Most of the women's self-esteem was very low and the institutional care simply reinforced those beliefs. Bundles of ill-fitting clothes were laid out every day, which included bras, knickers, crimplene dresses and cardigans, all previously worn by another person the day before.

Living together in cramped wards with 30 beds in a dormitory allowed no privacy whatsoever and most of the women became accustomed to dressing and undressing in front of each other. The degradation didn't stop there, because each woman was obliged to announce to the staff when they were menstruating so that it could be duly recorded in a menstruation book. Because of this, the women and staff used the phrase 'on the books' instead of more appropriate terms. I subsequently worked with women who moved from institutions over 20 years ago and they still used 'on the books' to describe their periods. The women had no choice but to report their menstruation, because it was their only way of getting sanitary wear. It was also a way of ensuring that nobody had become pregnant by not swallowing their contraceptive pill.

As you can imagine there was no choice of sanitary wear and sanitary towels with loops were provided that were to be worn with a belt. I recall that there were two sizes available, but these were very bulky and uncomfortable to wear and could be seen if the women wore trousers. Tampons were never offered to the women but I do not remember the reason why. I can only assume that these were more expensive to purchase and that it was believed that the women could not use them. I can remember offering pain relief to the women when they asked. However, I do not recall any of the women receiving advice on well women issues such as painful sexual intercourse, amenorrhoea, constant bleeding or irregular periods. Certainly, breast awareness and cervical screening were not offered. Generally, the medical support to the wards was by a psychiatrist who was usually male. I believe this factor alone stopped many women asking further questions and exploring their own sexuality.

In 1987 I left the institution to work in a six-bedded inpatient unit in a rural community in Devon. It was not until I left that I realised how awful life had been for the people I had worked with in the institutions. The smaller unit offered freedom of choice and treated each person as an individual. Unlike the institution, staff and residents shared toilets, crockery and cutlery. Mealtimes were a joint experience allowing for free flowing conversation. For the first time I felt that there was no barrier between staff and residents. Unconsciously I began to change my views and develop some of the work I am involved in today.

Introducing Jenna

I was a manager of a local support unit that offered six admission beds for assessment, treatment and support to clients and their families in the local community, when Jenna was admitted. Jenna's life story was very tragic and her case notes made sad reading. She had been born to a mildly learning disabled mother who was unable to manage with a new baby. The father was never mentioned in her records and she was quickly placed into care. Jenna was eventually fostered into a family where she was very much seen as the fostered child and providing an income to her foster parents. There was no record of Jenna's early years in the information in her files. She attended schools for the educationally subnormal, as they were called at that time, and moved around quite frequently because her foster father changed employment on a regular basis.

At the age of 17 Jenna's foster carers felt unable to continue to care for her and told her that she had to move out, as she was now an adult. This was the learning disability team's first contact with Jenna who, up until then, had led quite a sheltered life at home. Jenna was admitted to the local support unit for an assessment of her needs and wishes and to develop the skills and confidence to lead a more independent life. Jenna appeared to be a shy, immature young woman who was very unsure of herself and people around her.

After Jenna had been with us some months, she began to come out of her shell and I formed a very good relationship with her. This was helped by the relaxed atmosphere on the unit. The unit was small and allowed individuals the opportunity to become independent and the staff team were confident in standing back and letting this happen. This was a far cry from the institutional regime. Jenna also discovered that she loved to swim and the staff would often take her to the local pool. She quickly became quite an accomplished swimmer, which boosted her self-confidence immensely.

Up until this point Jenna and I had never touched on the subject of women's issues. Obviously, I had supported her with her menstruation and provided her with help in purchasing sanitary towels but I had not had any in-depth discussions with her about her body and the feelings she had about herself. That was until one day when Jenna asked to go swimming. As I knew she was menstruating I found myself saying that she could not go because she could not wear pads in the pool. 'Why not?' was her quick reply. I then found myself explaining that she could not swim unless she used tampons. Then I thought, 'God, who has the problem here?' I thought I had come a long way from my archaic, institutional upbringing and yet I was not prepared to explore the issue. Worst of all, most women, including myself, went swimming whilst menstruating, so why was I being obstructive and dismissive of Jenna? I concluded that the stark reality was that it was easier to be obstructive than to be constructive and to deal with the problem. I was quite happy to discuss menstruation but I realised that I had never looked at alternatives to using sanitary towels and, more poignantly, taught someone to use tampons. Jenna managed her periods independently and maintained good menstrual hygiene. She was able to choose appropriate sanitary towels for herself and coped well with their disposal. In fact, there was nothing to suggest that, with patience, sensitivity and time, Jenna could not be taught how to use tampons.

This now became very much my problem but how should I address it? Recently, there has been more written on the subject of menstruation (Rodgers, 2001). However, at the time, I was unable to find any literature on the subject. I felt I needed an in-depth, word-by-word format of how to teach someone. I recognised that this was a totally unrealistic expectation and I soon realised I would have to tailor my teaching to a pace and level that was acceptable to Jenna. She trusted me and relied on me to solve what to her, at the time, was a minor irritant and was stopping her from going swimming.

Eventually, I was able to find some valuable teaching aids. I took some pages from the Lifefacts pack (Stanfield & Downer, 1990) which I felt would give me a good pictorial description of a woman's anatomy and allow me to explain where the tampon was to be inserted. I also purchased various packets of tampons with Jenna so that she could choose which she would like and feel happy with. As with most feminine hygiene products there is so much choice available but they have slight differences. For example, some tampons have cardboard applicators and some do not. This may seem trivial but it was important for Jenna to be aware of both types in case she became confused when buying her own in the future. As soon as I began teaching Jenna about the application and insertion of a tampon it became clear that I had omitted the most vital information right at the beginning. I assumed that she was completely familiar with her own anatomy and knew common words such as vagina, fanny, pubic hair and anus. Although some people with learning disabilities might be familiar with those words, Jenna had no idea where they were on her body or what they meant. Having periods was something that happened to her each month but she had no knowledge of why and how they happened.

Rodgers (2001) described bringing a learning disabled woman's attention to the fact that menstruation means she is a woman and capable of bearing children. Sadly for Jenna, up until now, she had no concept of this at all. Suddenly I had opened a whole can of worms that had totally stretched my abilities as a nurse. Waterhouse & Metcalfe (1996) suggested that nurses felt embarrassed and inadequately trained to initiate discussion of sexuality matters with clients. Fortunately I had colleagues around me with more experience than myself who were able to direct and support me. Quite by chance, a colleague who had been teaching sex education to a couple had found an innovative way to explain the female anatomy to a woman who could not understand from pictures alone, where her reproductive organs were in her body. Whilst setting up the slide projector someone walked in front of the screen and had the slide projected onto themselves. With some slight modification my colleague went on to successfully teach the individual concerned.

I was able to use this approach with Jenna who was also unable to relate to what was underneath her skin and bone. The slide method enabled Jenna to see within herself. Sadly for Jenna she had not received any form of body awareness or basic sex education training in her life. She had picked up some terminology throughout her childhood that gave the impression that she was much more aware than she actually was. Wolfe & Blanchett (2000) stated that: 'information related to sexuality is often not made available to individuals with disabilities at any age due to the misperception that they are perpetual children'. Fairbairn (1995) said, 'people with learning disabilities have the right to be informed about sexuality and its place in human life as positively as possible'.

Although somewhat delayed, I decided it was not too late to teach Jenna more about sexuality because we had developed a good trusting relationship and she was a keen and interested student. However, I needed to concentrate on one area at a time and Jenna was desperate to swim every week. Using line drawings from the Lifefacts pack and projecting them onto a screen helped to show Jenna where things were in relation to her own body. I also used words that Jenna was happy and familiar with. I didn't feel it was necessary to use all the correct names and teach Jenna new words just for the sake of her sounding polite. Jenna chose 'fanny', which represented all her female genitalia and 'bum' for everything else. Jenna was a very private young woman and did not talk about her periods or use the words to describe her anatomy unless it was appropriate and she felt safe and comfortable. In the way Laws (1990) describes, Jenna was beginning to develop 'menstrual etiquette', whereby in white British culture menstruation remained hidden, especially from men.

Although Jenna was now beginning to realise where things were in her body, I felt I needed a further prompt to encourage her to use a tampon. A colleague had two cloth dolls that she had used to teach sex education. The dolls, one male and one female, stood about three feet high. They were fully clothed but these were removable and they had fully developed sexual organs underneath. The female doll had been used solely to teach menstrual care in the past and so I decided to use this approach with Jenna. Jenna immediately took to the doll, gave her a name and was happy to dress and undress her. I began slowly introducing the tampon to Jenna and showing her where to insert it into the doll. Although a little nervous at first Jenna was soon happy to insert the tampon into the doll herself. I left the doll with Jenna to enable her to practice in the privacy of her own room for a couple of days until she felt ready to move on. When I resumed teaching with Jenna I had to laugh as the doll had a new hairstyle and was wearing a scarf!

The next step was for Jenna to insert a tampon by herself. The doll's size and flexibility was ideal as it allowed Jenna to practise whilst holding the doll around her waist and bending slightly. She was then able to insert the tampon into the doll in very much the position that she would adopt herself. Jenna then moved on to using a tampon herself. To make it easier, I applied some vaseline to the end and I then left the room whilst Jenna inserted the tampon. Jenna called me in when she was happy and re-dressed. I checked with Jenna that the tampon was inserted in far enough by questioning her and ensuring that she could sit and walk comfortably. Jenna then took the tampon out and disposed of it appropriately. We practised this for a couple of days until she was totally confident.

Jenna was elated that she had achieved this herself and I was very proud of her. Using the doll proved to be highly successful and, without it, I was unsure if my training would have worked. The doll enabled Jenna to practise until she felt competent and allowed me to teach without ever having to cross the boundaries of invading Jenna's privacy. I never felt the need to see if the tampon was correctly inserted because I could watch her practise on the doll. Jenna was taught the importance of not wearing tampons for too long and the dangers of toxic shock syndrome. Jenna herself chose at that time to only use tampons when she went swimming. Jenna was involved in the whole care planning process and helped me to word her care plan.

The dolls are still used as a resource within the community team. I think they originally came as part of a teaching package from the Brook Advisory Service. Being resourceful and ingenious is part and parcel of being a learning disability nurse. As nurses we are often looking for elaborate resources to use as teaching aids when, in fact, my nurse training taught me to concentrate mainly on communication skills. If there is little or no communication between student and teacher resources are of minimal use. We must also recognise our own limitations and be prepared to ask others for help.

Growing up

I did not set out to teach a sexuality package to Jenna. Indeed, she had been admitted for assessment with a view to a quick discharge into the community, once the consultant was happy with her progress. Six months had passed since her admission and Jenna had become a different person. She was more outgoing, confident and aware of her own sexuality. Grigg (2001) cites Llewelyn Jones (1986) as saying:

> 'Sexuality is the sum of a person's inherited make-up, knowledge, experiences, attitudes and behaviour as he or she relates to being a man or woman.'

During the period of Jenna's admission the staff team consisted of ten females and two males. The majority of female staff were of a similar age to Jenna and, looking back, were a great influence on her.

Jenna had experienced quite a sheltered upbringing with older foster parents. All of a sudden, Jenna had to live in a busy unit with five other people, with various care needs, of both genders and 12 different care staff. Jenna was popular with most of the staff. Like any other adolescent, Jenna enjoyed dressing up, having her hair and make-up done and generally being made a fuss of. The staff shared their interests in music, fashion, beauty and make-up with her. Murray *et al.* (2001) recognised the fact that the staff team can have other influences on the lives of people with learning disabilities by stating that staff in residential care play:

> 'an integral role in influencing clients' daily behaviour and have a significant impact on many aspects of sexuality. These issues are of primary importance to the rights and empowerment of people with learning disabilities.'

This was evident to the staff team on the unit. It seemed to us that Jenna had done a lot of growing up whilst on the unit. She had gained insight into her sexuality and her body by learning about menstrual hygiene. The staff had also helped to raise Jenna's self-esteem by encouraging her to take more pride in herself. Jenna enjoyed pampering herself, choosing smart clothes, having long bubble baths and wearing make-up. These are things we take for granted but she had not had an opportunity to experience them until now.

However, as Jenna's self-awareness grew, so did her frustrations. Jenna began to form inappropriate relationships with the two male members of staff in the unit. We noticed that she had become very flirtatious and overfamiliar and began asking questions of a sexual nature. The male staff were very anxious to support Jenna through this. However, they did not want to be put in a position whereby they could be accused of encouraging her. As manager of the unit during this time I took the decision that no male member of staff should work a shift on their own. Paparestis (2001) cites Bowlby (1988), who emphasised the importance of attachment and how it can develop a secure base for an individual.

> 'If relationships with peers are poor, there will be pressure on relationships with staff, which can make staff feel defensive. Staff attitudes play a huge part in what is seen and addressed, something very much influenced by our own thoughts, views and feelings. We need to look at ourselves as part of this picture, and also consider the meaning of our relationship with clients sensitively without being burdened by guilt.'

I began to reflect on what was causing Jenna to form these relationships. I thought that one reason was that she wanted a boyfriend of her own, as some of her peers in the unit had formed relationships at the day centre and most of the staff had partners. I also thought that Jenna had not yet learned that relationships could take on different forms. For example, Jenna could have been transferring her need to be loved and cared for onto the male members of staff. One staff member seemed to take on a 'father figure' role in Jenna's eyes. I wondered whether her poor relationship with her foster father and his inability to display affection towards her made her crave the attention of men. Furthermore, because she had not experienced a nurturing, caring relationship between a father and daughter, Jenna had little idea how to relate towards other men. As Lesseliers (1999) wrote, 'the circumstances of people's lives shape their perceptions of sexuality and relationships'.

I decided to work with Jenna to explore the different relationships in her life that had been so difficult for her because of her upbringing and her transient lifestyle with the foster family. Teaching friendships and social skills with Jenna became the hardest aspect of my work with her. I think I found it so complex because Jenna had nothing to relate to. The closest she had come to having a caring, nurturing relationship was with the staff in the unit. In Jenna's eyes we were becoming the family she had never had. Looking back at that area of my work with her, I did not use any particular model of care with Jenna and I think I failed to recognise my lack of knowledge on this subject. On reflection, perhaps I should have referred Jenna to another professional, such as a psychologist, and not relied so heavily on the trusting relationship that Jenna and I had formed together. Having said that, Jenna did not try to form any further inappropriate relationships within the staff team. Whether this was a direct result of the work we did together or a natural change in Jenna I will never know.

Moving on

'People with a learning disability must be prepared for the adult world. Their vulnerability means that they need more than just a sex education programme. Coping with possible sexual exploitation is about knowing your rights, having the chance to experience relationships and knowing how to react and behave, with them. Ignorance is not bliss, it is dangerous.' (Carr, 1995)

Jenna eventually found a community placement with a local landlady and her family. The landlady's husband worked away from home for long periods at a time on an oil rig and Jenna became good company for her landlady. At the same time Jenna found work at a large clothing factory nearby. The change in Jenna was apparent almost immediately and she became vocal and rebellious. She was also quite indignant and almost embarrassed to have to associate with professionals when she was with her new friends. Jenna had work colleagues to mix with and this new peer group had now become very influential in her life. Jenna started smoking, going to pubs and clubs and was looking to have a great time.

Fortunately, Jenna maintained some contact with the learning disability team and myself. On one of the visits I made she asked for contraceptive advice and she made it clear that she did not want a baby. I felt flattered that Jenna still valued our relationship. I had some concerns over her new lifestyle which I was unable to change; all I could do was to sit back and be there if she needed me. Prior to visiting her doctor, Jenna and I looked at all the alternatives available to her. I got examples of all the contraceptives for her to touch and look at and explained what they were and how they were used. Jenna quickly dismissed the coil and diaphragm and chose to have a progestogen injection because she felt she might forget to take the contraceptive pill. I explained the likely side effects of this, in particular the weight gain and the lack of menstruation.

At that time, I was unsure if Jenna was already in a relationship or whether she had someone in mind. I thought that she had been encouraged by her friends to go on the pill and that they had probably talked about using it or she had seen them take it. I was pleased that she had made her own informed choice about contraception and had not chosen the pill simply to follow her friends' example. Jenna and I talked about casual sex and the importance of being safe. I felt Jenna had decided that she would have sex sooner rather than later, even though she did not have a regular boyfriend. Paparestis (2001) stated that:

> 'a sexual relationship could be seen to offer status and allow a woman to feel valued and like other "normal" women in society, and no longer different; this may be an additional motive to all the other reasons for which people engage in relationships. Previous losses in relationships may also act as additional pressures for sexual relationships, in which they appear to be seeking a significant other to curb their loneliness and compensate for the losses they have experienced.'

Therefore, when establishing a way of working with an individual it is important to keep an open mind and listen to their agenda rather than be led by our own. Inadvertently, I may have deviated from this advice. I was very concerned that Jenna was engaging in sex for all the wrong reasons and I felt very protective towards her. Although Jenna had probably grown up over the past two years and was able to give consent, there remained a naivety about her that made her seem vulnerable at times. Jenna was not prepared to talk to me any further on this occasion about healthy sex or using condoms to protect her from sexually transmitted diseases and for the first time my advice fell on deaf ears.

I did not see Jenna until her next contraceptive injection was due some months later. Jenna still chose to have someone to accompany her whilst attending the doctor's surgery. I felt quite relieved that she still felt comfortable with my support. Jenna talked about a relationship she had with a man at the factory. She appeared quite confused about it, as he would only see her on certain days. Their sexual relationship was confined to his car and he never offered to take her home or out for a drink. Jenna was obviously very fond of this man because he showed her affection and made her feel wanted. Jenna had enough insight to realise that something in this relationship was not right and I felt that, rather than tell her to stop seeing him and tell her she was being used, it was better for her to work through it with me.

I based my discussions with her on what McCarthy & Thompson (1993) call the '3Rs', which are rights, responsibilities and risks. Jenna and I talked about relationships and how she imagined a relationship should be between a man and a woman. Jenna described wanting to be taken out, being made a fuss of and actually sleeping with a man all night. Sexual intercourse was not a priority for Jenna and, when she compared her ideal relationship to the relationship she was in, she began to see what was happening to her. This is highlighted by McCarthy & Thompson (2000) who stated, 'When women with learning disabilities become sexual adults, they don't often get what they want and they often get what they don't want.' Jenna lacked the confidence to tell the man that she did not want this type of relationship. Although I explored with Jenna her becoming more assertive, it seemed to me that this relationship was more important to Jenna than no relationship at all. She was not prepared to lose it and be on her own again. Murray *et al.* (2001) stated that:

> 'Disadvantages in communication and negotiation skills, difficulties in assertiveness and the legacy of social disincentives for sexual behaviour, all create serious obstacles for sexual expression by people with learning disabilities.'

Seeing Jenna in this type of relationship really made me question my own abilities to support her. By using my supervision I was able to discuss my concerns and put my feelings into perspective. The conclusion being that Jenna was a consenting adult and that together we had looked at changing things. Jenna did not agree to changing any part of the relationship and did not want her partner involved. It is sometimes very difficult to stand back and watch from a distance when your instincts are screaming at you to intervene. Jenna was clear in making an informed choice of her own. People in the local community were unaware of Jenna's mild learning disability or my involvement with her.

Jenna's relationship with the man at the factory ended after someone reported them having sex in the car. They were both reprimanded by the factory manager, but Jenna coped well with this and the loss of the relationship. Jenna was lucky to keep her job. However, I did wonder if all the other staff would have been quite so fortunate if they were seen in broad daylight having sex in the factory grounds. Jenna and I talked about appropriate places for her to have sex. Her landlady was happy for Jenna to bring a boyfriend home. Understandably, she did not want Jenna coming home with lots of different men, as there were young children in the house.

The situation remained stable until Jenna lost her job at the factory. Jenna had been taking a lot of time off sick and was not working when she was there. Apparently, Jenna had developed relationships with quite a few men at the factory and was seeing them when they were on opposite shifts to her own. It seemed that Jenna had become very promiscuous and certain men seemed quite willing to take advantage of this. Jenna did not seem to care where she actually had sex or if anyone saw her. There were reports of her having sex in the bushes near to the factory and in the local park. This raised several concerns for me. The UKCC (1998) gave advice to nurses on the subject of sexuality that stated that, 'you must allow clients to express their sexuality appropriately but this must be balanced against the risk of abuse or exploitation'.

Apart from the professional issues, to say I wasn't disappointed or upset with Jenna's behaviour would have been a lie. I was finding it difficult to accept the change in her more than the actual casual relationships she had chosen. If Jenna had chosen to have these relationships in private nobody would ever have known. Therefore, it was important to address the issue of privacy before the police arrested her. Jenna had not been able to take men back to her house because her landlady's husband was at home permanently. I learned that he was a very domineering man whom Jenna found very intimidating and who reminded her of her foster father. I thought that this situation could be easily resolved if Jenna got a small flat of her own. Jenna and I discussed the dangers of multiple partners and the risks of sexually transmitted diseases and of abuse. Living on her own would give Jenna the ability to be independent but, at the same time, would put her at risk of being exploited by one or more of the men she knew. I encouraged Jenna to visit the local family planning centre so that she had the opportunity to talk about her sexual health to someone other than myself. As I was unsure of who Jenna's partners were I felt it was necessary for her to take the responsibility of obtaining and using condoms. Jenna assured me that she used them regularly.

> 'This reflects a general attitude that women are targeted as being responsible for contraception and safer sex precautions, despite the fact that both sexes are equally present in the heterosexual activity.' (McCarthy, 1996)

By this time, I was based with the community learning disability team and I was able to visit Jenna weekly. She coped well with her newly found independence. The flat was clean and there had been no more public displays of a sexual nature. Jenna had no permanent relationship, although sex remained a very important part of her life. I am unsure how things would have developed had things gone differently for her during her childhood. Jenna evidently craved affection from men. I had no doubts that some of her sexual experiences had been very negative: 'Women with learning disabilities tend to be the passive partners, their sexual pleasure is conspicuous only by its absence.'

(McCarthy, 1996). I am sure Jenna had felt obliged to go along with what her partners wanted sexually. Somehow I now felt this had changed and that as her sexual experiences grew she was clearer about what she wanted from a relationship.

The most recent piece of work I completed with Jenna was to accompany her for her first cervical smear. Ager & Littler (1998) stated that:

> 'Early detection of problems through screening services is an important feature of sexual health. Cervical screening is used to detect pre-cancerous changes, so that treatment can be offered to prevent invasive cervical cancer. Breast screening is used to detect early cancers.'

I have been very involved in the cervical screening process since I became a qualified smear taker having completed the Marie Curie Cervical Screening course, which gave me further insight into the whole procedure (Wilkins, 2000). Pearson *et al.* (1998) discovered that only a quarter of the eligible learning disabled women in this area had undergone screening in the previous five years compared to 82% of the rest of the eligible population. Along with a group of other professionals I helped to produce a health awareness pack, using real models to show cervical and breast screening. The easy to read format and colour photographs enabled Jenna to have an understanding of the procedure and what to expect. Jenna now had a good perception of her own body and knew where the speculum was to be inserted. She had visited the practice nurse on previous occasions and was familiar with the surgery setting. However, I felt it was important for Jenna to book a double appointment so that she could have her smear taken without being rushed and allow her time to ask questions. It is most important that learning disabled women attend mainstream primary care services wherever possible.

Piecing it all together

The World Health Organization (1986) defined sexual health as:

> 'a capacity to enjoy and control sexual and reproductive behaviour in accordance with a social and personal ethic. Freedom from fear, shame, guilt, false belief and other psychological factors inhibiting sexual response and impairing sexual relationships and freedom that interfere with sexual and reproductive functions.'

Throughout Jenna's story I have discussed experiences that we shared together. I had not originally set out to work through so much with Jenna nor did I ever profess to know the answers to all the challenges she faced me with. The sexual health of women with learning disabilities should not be a one-off piece of work however able they may be. Women need continuing information about their bodies as they mature and experience different relationships in their lives. Sex education should go further than teaching women about contraceptives and personal hygiene. Women need to be encouraged to feel comfortable with their bodies and how they function. They need to know about friendships, respect for others and how to remain safe. Women also need to know that relationships fail and that they may not always live up to their expectations. As teachers of sexual health issues we must be prepared to address our own beliefs and acknowledge issues that we may feel prejudiced about. We must be aware and comfortable with our own sexuality.

Since gaining more knowledge in women's health issues I realise it is very important for learning disability nurses to continue to raise other professionals' awareness of the importance of sexual health and screening for learning disabled women and how not to allow assumptions to be made that they do not require a service.

References

Ager, J. & Littler, J. (1998) Sexual Health for people with learning disabilities. *Nursing Standard*, **13**(2), 34–9.

Bowlby, J. (1998) *A secure base: clinical applications of attachment theory*. Routledge, London.

Carr, L.T. (1995) Sexuality and people with learning disabilities. *British Journal of Nursing*, **4**(19), 1135–41.

Fairbairn, G. (1995) *Sexuality, learning difficulties and doing what's right*. David Fulton, London.

Grigg, E. (2001) Sexuality matters. *Learning Disability Practice*, **3**(5), 16–21.

Laws, S. (1990) *Issues of Blood. The politics of menstruation*. Macmillan, Basingstoke.

Lesseliers, J. (1999) A right to sexuality? *British Journal of Learning Disability*, **27**, 137–40.

Llewelyn Jones, A. (1986) *Understanding sexuality*. Oxford University Press, Oxford.

McCarthy, M. (1996) The sexual support needs of people with learning disabilities: a profile of those referred for sex education. *Sexuality and Disability*, **14**(4), 265–77.

McCarthy, M. & Thompson, D. (1993) *Sex and The 3Rs*. Pavilion Publishing, Brighton.

McCarthy, M. & Thompson, D. (2000) Becoming a sexual adult. *ACT Bulletin*, July 2000, 6–11.

Murray, J., Macdonald, R. & Levenson, V. (2001) Sexuality: Policies, Beliefs and Practice. *Tizard Learning Disability Review*, **6**(1), 29–34.

Paparestis, C. (2001) Women with Learning Disabilities – Experiencing their sexuality in a healthy way. *Tizard Learning Disability Review*, **6**(1), 22–4.

Pearson, V., Davis, C., Ruoff, C. & Dyer, J. (1998) Only one quarter of women with a learning disability in Exeter have cervical screening. *British Medical Journal*, **316**.

Rodgers, J. (2001) The experience and management of menstruation for women with learning disabilities. *Tizard Learning Disability Review*, **6**(1), 36–43.

Stanfield, J. & Downer, A. (1990) *Lifefacts pack (sexuality); Essential information about life for persons with special needs*. James Stanfield Company, New York.

UKCC (1988) *Guidelines for Mental Health and Learning Disabilities Nursing.* UKCC, London.

Waterhouse, J. & Metcalfe, M. (1996) Attitudes towards nurses discussing sexual concerns with patients. *Journal of Advanced Nursing*, **16**, 1048–54.

Wilkins, J. (2000) Pioneering Spirit. *Learning Disability Practice*, **3**(1), 4–8.

Wolfe, P. & Blanchett, W. (2000) The right to sexual expression. *TASH Newsletter*, May 2000, 5–7.

World Health Organization Regional Office for Europe (1986) *Concepts for sexual health.* WHO, Copenhagen.

Further reading

Burns, J. (2000) Gender identity and women with learning disabilities, the third sex. *Clinical Psychology Forum*, 137, 11–15.

McCarthy, M. (1999) *Sexuality and women with learning disabilities.* Jessica Kingsley Publishers, London.

McCarthy, M. & Thompson, D. (1997) A prevalence study of sexual abuse of adults with intellectual disabilities referred for sex education. *Journal of Applied Research in Intellectual Disability*, **10**(2), 105–24.

Chapter 11

A shock to the system: improving encounters with acute health care

Adrian Jones

A sense of injustice

On reflection, becoming a learning disability nurse was inevitable for me. As a child I had a small group of friends with whom I played regularly. Amongst these friends was a boy with a learning disability who had a number of medical problems. Although we were conscious of the fact that he was often unable to play because he was unwell, he was otherwise a regular member of our gang who shared with us a passion for watching and playing football on the street outside his house. However, I also recall as a child that I was frequently angered by the attitude of other boys from the estate who ridiculed him. My friends and I were often involved in fights to defend his 'honour'. The feelings of anger and injustice that I felt then have stayed with me throughout my life and have played a major role in shaping my beliefs, both personally and professionally, about society and how it treats those who have disabilities. I can certainly recall making a conscious decision that if life ever provided me with an opportunity to do something positive for disabled people, then I would endeavour to do my best to make a difference in some way.

Another important influence on me was the voluntary work I undertook as a young adult with both my parish church and the local branch of the British Red Cross Society. This brought me into regular contact with a number of adults with learning disabilities and I came to realise that I quite enjoyed working with them. I began to explore employment opportunities for work with people with disabilities, although at the time I was not thinking of people with learning disabilities. The work with the Red Cross raised the possibility of a career as a nurse, although I had no idea at the time that there was a branch of nursing devoted to people with learning disabilities. However, once I found this out, I knew this was the career path I needed to follow.

During my career as a nurse there have been times when I have found myself frustrated and angered by a society that disadvantages and discriminates against people who have disabilities. Like many people who trained a decade or so ago, my first staff nurse post was in an old long-stay hospital. My first ward was home to a group of adults, some of whom were quite elderly, who had profound learning disabilities. The environment was sparse, with little or no privacy, despite the best efforts of the staff. The facilities were basic and I recall the frustration of waiting several months for the repair of a commode chair at a time when the local general hospital launched an appeal, and rapidly achieved its target, for raising £250 000 to buy a body scanner. Whilst I recognised there was a need for the scanner, this seemed to highlight the different value that society places on different groups of individuals.

As a student nurse I can also remember taking one of the hospital residents for a haircut. As we approached, the barber saw us coming and greeted us with a cheery smile at the door.

'Sorry, mate,' he announced, 'I'm closed.'

I did not believe him, so I walked around the corner and waited a few moments. To my disgust, when I walked past the shop a couple of minutes later, not only was the shop open, but there was a new customer waiting. On another occasion I sat in a roadside café having a meal with colleagues and two teenagers with multiple disabilities, after a day out at a theme park. We were made to feel very unwelcome by the staff who hinted that they would prefer it if we did not order a dessert, as they did not want us to stay much longer. They suggested that the physical appearance of the teenagers was putting off potential customers from entering the café. These two events left a lasting impression on me and filled me with a number of emotions. In the first instance, I was angered at the blatant discrimination displayed by others. Second, I felt ashamed and embarrassed to be a member of a society that could be so willing to treat fellow human beings in such a derogatory manner.

Unfortunately, it is not only members of the general public who air such prejudicial views. To my continuing dismay I still come across fellow professionals who offer negative opinions about people with learning disabilities. It is a source of great concern to me that people with learning disabilities may be dependent for their care and support upon people who hold such discriminatory views.

As a learning disability nurse now employed in an acute hospital setting, I believe that it is important to raise the awareness of care staff to the needs of people with learning disabilities in order that they receive a level of care and support that is appropriate to their needs. Coming into hospital is a stressful time for any patient. If that patient happens to have a learning disability then additional preparation may be necessary that is both informed and sensitive. In the United States, Criscione *et al.* (1995) showed that the inpatient experience, discharge and aftercare of individuals with learning disabilities could be improved if a specialist nurse in learning disability managed the admission and discharge. Unfortunately, I believe that people with learning disabilities and their carers have tended to receive hospital care that falls short of an acceptable standard. This is in spite of the fact that services for people with learning disabilities have undergone considerable scrutiny over the past three decades. This scrutiny has shown, in particular, that people with learning disabilities receive a poor service from mainstream health services (Department of Health, 1995; Kerr *et al.*, 1996).

The new White Paper for learning disability, *Valuing People* (Department of Health, 2001), acknowledges that people with learning disabilities are among the most socially excluded and vulnerable groups in society. The White Paper has set a number of ambitious targets to ensure that the necessary help and support is available to foster independence and improve the quality of services. Many of these targets build on previous guidance and good practice statements. For example, *Signposts for Success* (Department of Health, 1998) emphasised that people with learning disabilities should be helped to use the full range of health services. This could include securing extra resources to set up dedicated clinics or training to build additional competence and confidence in working with people with learning disabilities and their carers. The document *Once a Day* (Department of Health, 1999) added to this by giving specific advice to general practitioners (GPs) on making their practices more accessible to people with learning disabilities.

Routine procedures

It is against this background that I would like to introduce Julie. Julie was 37 years of age and had a severe learning disability. She was tall, strong, of stocky build and in general good health. She lived with her parents in a rural area and attended a day centre for adults three days a week. Julie did not communicate with speech but was able to make her needs known to her parents through vocalisations and facial expressions. Her parents were quite elderly and her father had an industrial-related illness which meant that he had not been well for some time. Therefore, Julie's mother became her main carer, though her older brother was very supportive and contributed significantly towards her care by helping with transport to respite breaks. I found out from her parents that Julie did not cope well with being in unfamiliar environments or being with unfamiliar people. Unfortunately for Julie, a minor health problem that she had had for a while had suddenly become more acute and the only way it could be resolved was by surgery under general anaesthetic. Although the operation was relatively routine, it was not available at her local hospital. Therefore, Julie was admitted to the surgical ward where I worked as a staff nurse.

One of the difficulties frequently encountered by nursing staff working in hospital is that they are often unaware that a patient has learning disabilities until the person actually arrives on the ward. It is not unusual for the referral letter from the GP to make no mention of this fact. Even if the referral contains this information it is rare for it to be communicated to the staff who are providing the day-to-day care. Therefore, it is very difficult for staff to plan and coordinate effective care in advance of the person entering hospital.

Julie had been referred to the hospital several weeks before her attendance for surgery and had been reviewed at an outpatient appointment. Her GP referral letter stated that Julie had a severe learning disability but no other details were provided except for her medical history. Following her attendance at the outpatient appointment, she was listed for surgery as a day case. The first time the ward staff received any information about Julie happened the afternoon before Julie was admitted when the theatre list for the next day was delivered to the ward. The only information given on the list was Julie's name, sex, date of birth, her place on the operating list and the fact that she had a severe learning disability. Such little information is hardly the ideal preparation for either the staff or the patient.

Julie arrived on the ward at 7.30 in the morning on the day of her surgery, accompanied by her mother and brother. They had travelled about 35 miles to get to the hospital, so this had meant an early start for them. By the time they arrived on the ward it was clear that Julie was already quite agitated and her mother was also showing signs of strain. The family was greeted by staff and shown to a single room at the end of the ward. The first thing I discovered when checking the theatre list was that Julie was not scheduled to go down to theatre until the early afternoon. Julie's mother had been told to wake her early and give her a drink and something light to eat before they had set off for the hospital. Julie, still not fully awake at the time, had accepted the drink but refused anything to eat before they left home. It had been too early for Julie when her mother offered her something to eat but it was now eight o'clock and she was hungry. She could see and smell the breakfast that was being brought round for the other patients, so why couldn't she have some?

Tensions mount

As the morning wore on, Julie became increasingly unsettled and agitated. She was hungry, thirsty and frustrated at being confined to a ward area with nothing to do. It was impossible to explain to Julie why she could not have anything to eat or drink but all she wanted to do was satisfy her hunger and thirst. The situation was made worse by her being in a strange environment and being approached by people who she did not know. Julie's mother, a small, thin lady, confessed to me that she was very anxious about how the day would unfold. Julie's brother, a large, strong-looking man, did not say much but sat in the room with Julie and her mother and read a book for much of the time. The room that they occupied was a spacious one and I explained to them that they were free to wander around the ward but not leave the ward until the anaesthetist and doctors had visited Julie. I contacted the doctor and was told that they could come to see her within an hour. However, the anaesthetist was not in the hospital and could not see her until lunch-time.

When I admitted Julie, the first problem I encountered was trying to record her temperature, pulse, blood pressure and her weight. It quickly became apparent that she was not going to let me or anyone else go near her. She became distressed when I approached and she shouted out and tried to push me away. Julie was very strong and I quickly realised why her brother had accompanied her. Although it is routine to record a patient's observations on admission, I was not too concerned about taking them at that moment. I judged that she was in good health and there would be other opportunities to make observations. However, to my dismay, Julie's brother had other ideas and he leapt to his feet and tried to make her comply with my wishes by struggling with her. Obviously, this made the situation worse and I felt that any attempt to establish a trusting relationship with Julie had been seriously damaged.

I felt annoyed and frustrated that Julie had become upset and more distressed than she needed to be. I felt that forward planning could have helped prepare Julie, her mother and also the rest of the nursing staff. Even a simple measure, such as putting her on the theatre list for the morning, would have meant that she would have avoided a distressing wait. It would also have meant that she would have the afternoon to recover and every chance of returning home the same day as her surgery. I was also growing more uncomfortable at the degree of physical restraint practised by Julie's brother.

By the time the anaesthetist came onto the ward to see her, Julie was still very upset. She paced the room and cried out. She would not be comforted and, by now, I was extremely doubtful that we would be able to get her to calm down sufficiently to get her to theatre for surgery. The anaesthetist was undaunted and prescribed a premedication that would hopefully sedate Julie and allow her to settle. During the morning we had eventually been able to weigh Julie, so the appropriate dose could be calculated. I first attempted to persuade Julie to take the medication by relying mainly on non-threatening body posture. Despite this, it became clear that Julie did not trust me, or my colleagues. In the end, Julie's mother placed the medicine in a drinking cup that was similar to one that Julie was familiar with at home. As I observed the situation from outside the room, Julie took the medication from her mother. Although the decision to give Julie her medication in this way was the responsibility of her mother, it was uncomfortable for me, as a professional, to be seen to be complying with it. In 2001, the UKCC issued guidance for all nurses on this very issue. The UKCC set out the circumstances when it could be acceptable to conceal medication.

After a while, Julie became drowsy and less vocal than she had been previously. I gave her mother a theatre gown and left her to get Julie undressed and into her gown. I had begun to think that the situation might turn out all right. I could see Julie fighting against sleep, although she shouted out occasionally. However, things quickly took a turn for the worst. Unfortunately, the premedication chosen by the anaesthetist can have a number of side effects and, in some people, this can include unpleasant hallucinations as well as nausea and vomiting. Shortly before Julie was due to go to theatre, she began to retch quite forcibly. This carried on for some time and she became agitated and distressed once again. The anaesthetist was contacted over the telephone and, to my amazement, requested that I administer a further small dose of the medication she had already been given, together with an anti-emetic. I explained that I would be happy to administer something to stop the retching but I was not willing to sedate Julie any further. I stated that I felt that this would be unfair to her in her present state and I thought it unlikely that she would take any more medication. The anaesthetist agreed to come to the ward to review the situation.

Despite our best efforts, Julie would not take any further medication. Therefore, after discussing the situation with Julie's mother, brother, nursing staff and the surgeon, the operation was cancelled. Sadly, it proved impossible to persuade Julie to take anything for the sickness but the retching stopped in the early evening. Julie was not well enough to go home that night and stayed in hospital with her mother. This was obviously a source of great inconvenience and came at the end of a stressful day. Happily, by morning, Julie had recovered enough to go home. However, without careful planning, everyone felt that we were doomed to repeat this unsatisfactory experience.

Service-centred systems

Undoubtedly, some people with learning disabilities have been served well by mainstream health services. However, my experience as a learning disability and general nurse, as well as a wealth of research evidence, suggest that Julie's experience is not uncommon. People with learning disabilities are more likely to experience a much greater range and intensity of health problems than the general population (Department of Health, 1995). At the same time, evidence suggests that people with learning disabilities are living longer, a fact that may bring them into greater contact with acute health services (Fryers, 1987). The move away from hospital to community based forms of care has also brought with it an emphasis on the use of mainstream health services. Unfortunately, these trends have not been matched by action within both specialist services for people with learning disabilities as well as mainstream health services.

Looking back on Julie's experience, I was determined that lessons could be learned from the situation. One of the main problems with the service I worked in was that it was service-centred rather than patient-centred. Although the service had managed to achieve a great deal for many people, it operated mainly for the convenience of the people working in the system rather than those who accessed it. This was true in Julie's case but, with a little more flexibility and advanced planning, I began to think that her experience and the outcome could have been completely different.

My thoughts coincided with the publication of documents from the Department of Health, such as *Signposts for Success* (Department of Health, 1998), that emphasised the need for mainstream health services to improve their access for people with learning disabilities. Fortunately, in the hospital I worked in, managers were sympathetic to the need to improve the situation but I still had to lobby them at every opportunity to do something to improve access for people with learning disabilities. Eventually, a review group was established to explore the situation and experiences of people with learning disabilities and to make recommendations for change. As a learning disability nurse, I quickly became involved in the group. Our first task included producing a brief report for the group on my observations of the experiences of people with learning disabilities.

Later, the review group carried out a number of audits that were designed to gain the views of people with learning disabilities and their carers, about the service they had received. In particular, questions focused on areas such as admission planning; quality of information; communication with professionals; consent and confidentiality; the hospital environment, including comfort, meals and choice and, finally, the discharge planning process. A second audit tool was used to gain the views of informal and professional carers of people with learning disabilities. The results were undertaken over a three-month period and were used to provide a benchmark of current service delivery. For a nurse whose job had been to work with individuals day in and day out, it felt a little precarious to be contemplating and recommending such far-reaching proposals. However, I also found it exciting to use my knowledge of learning disability in new ways. In this way, I could potentially benefit hundreds of people with learning disabilities and their families.

The results of the audit, together with other information and the views of the review group, produced a number of recommendations. For example, one of the main areas of complaint was poor communication. Therefore, a new GP referral form was devised specifically for people with learning disabilities. This would provide the hospital with some basic information about the person that would not only include the person's medical history but other information such as their home and carer situation and details about professionals who support the person. Information about the new referral form has been disseminated through the practice managers at GP surgeries in the area. Upon receipt of the referral form, medical secretaries attach a plain coloured sticker to the cover of the person's notes to indicate that a person has a learning disability.

One of the key areas that I have been involved in has been the development of a learning disability assessment questionnaire. The nursing documentation that was being used did not allow for the depth of information needed to develop comprehensive, person-centred plans for people with learning disabilities while in hospital. The assessment questionnaire is posted to the patient with their first outpatient's appointment date and is designed to be completed by the person with a learning disability or their carer, prior to attending hospital. If information had been available about Julie prior to her arriving on the ward that morning, then the staff could have developed a plan based around her individual needs.

Another part of the process is to encourage the person, whenever possible, to attend the hospital for pre-clerking a week or so before admission. This has many advantages for all concerned. For example, the person could spend some time looking around the ward and meeting some of the people who will be providing their care. It would also offer the carer the chance to make contact with care staff on the ward. This visit can also offer the opportunity for the person to meet the doctor and anaesthetist. This could help highlight and resolve potential problems prior to admission. Almost all of the questions that need to be asked about the person's medical history could be asked at this meeting. Where appropriate, the anaesthetist could arrange for the person to go home with a mild sedating premedication. It may be better for the person to take this medication in the familiar surroundings of their own home thus taking the edge off their anxiety when they are eventually admitted. Some of the review group are now working on producing patient information in formats that will be easily understood. For example, this could include audio or video tapes that could be borrowed at the pre-admission visit.

If all of these innovations had been in place for Julie and her family, I am sure that she would have had a less stressful experience. With the information provided on the GP referral form, I could have made contact with either a community learning disability nurse or social worker and asked them to visit the family prior to admission. Any questions or issues could then have been passed on to the ward staff.

Another key area being addressed by the work of the review group is staff training. In Julie's case I felt very strongly that some staff, particularly the anaesthetist, did not have sufficient insight into Julie's needs. Slevin & Sines (1996) confirmed that some staff in acute hospital settings could develop negative attitudes towards people with learning disabilities. They also demonstrated that these attitudes could be changed through the intervention of a specialist in learning disability such as a learning disability nurse. In refusing to give further prescribed medication, I felt that it was my professional duty to act as an advocate for Julie and prevent any further distress. In my opinion, the anaesthetist did not act in a deliberately discriminatory way but simply displayed a lack of understanding that may have been the result of a lack of knowledge of people with learning disabilities.

In order to develop positive attitudes and values, nurses and other appropriate healthcare staff were invited to attend a basic disability awareness day. A two-day workshop with more specific information on the needs of people with learning disabilities is being planned. It is hoped that every member of staff attending this workshop will develop their own individual learning plan that will form part of their continuing professional development. Another area of change planned is to identify link roles in learning disability amongst staff in areas such as theatre and recovery, day care and other directorates such as medicine and surgery.

Conclusion

Changes in working practices are being introduced gradually. For example, people with learning disabilities will be offered longer appointment time slots. They will be first to be seen in outpatients' clinics with access to quiet waiting areas and minimal waiting times. It is also planned that people with learning disabilities, where appropriate, will be first on theatre lists and their care will be planned so that they have as short a stay as possible in hospital. Carers' issues are already being addressed with the development of facilities to support carers to stay with patients in hospital. Giving carers an option of whether to stay or not is an issue I feel very strongly about, having worked in areas where great pressure has been applied to carers to get them to stay and undertake virtually all of the care of the individual whilst they are in hospital. Although some carers are only to happy to participate in the care of the person, it is important that hospital staff do not assume that this will happen in every case.

References

Criscione, T., Walsh, K.K. & Kastner, T.A. (1995) An evaluation of care coordination in controlling inpatient hospital utilisation of people with developmental disabilities. *Mental Retardation*, **33**(6), 364–73.

Department of Health (1995) *The Health of the Nation for People with Learning Disabilities*. Department of Health, London.

Department of Health (1998) *Signposts for Success*. Department of Health, London.

Department of Health (1999) *Once a Day*. Department of Health, London.

Department of Health (2001) *Valuing People: A New Strategy for Learning Disability for the 21st Century*. Department of Health, London.

Fryers, T. (1987) Epidemiological issues in mental retardation. *Journal of Mental Deficiency Research*, **31**, 365–84.

Kerr, M., Dunstan, F. & Thapar, A. (1996) Attitudes of general practitioners to caring for people with learning disability. *British Journal of General Practice*, **46**, 92–4.

Slevin, E. & Sines, D. (1996) Attitudes of nurses in a general hospital towards people with learning disabilities: influences of contact and graduate-non-graduate status, a comparative study. *Journal of Advanced Nursing*, **24**, 1116–26.

United Kingdom Central Council (2001) *UKCC Position Statement on the Covert Administration of Medicines – Disguising Medicines in Food and Drink*. UKCC, London.

Chapter 12

Getting life under control: managing risks from epilepsy

Rebecca Welsh

Defining moments

At the age of four I attended a school where children with disabilities were integrated into the classes. I suppose that was progressive for 1978 but, to me, it was normal. My next introduction to people with disabilities happened when I began working in the field of outdoor education. Initially, I worked with schoolchildren but then moved to an outdoor centre that specialised in activity holidays for people with special needs. There were two defining moments from this period that set me on my way into nursing. The first was an encounter with a young man who spoke using an electronic communicator. When I first met him I have to confess that I judged him by his disability and made assumptions about his quality of life and abilities. During the week he communicated his basic needs, which I was able to meet but, towards the end of the week, he summoned me, activated his computer, and told an extremely funny and very risqué joke. It dawned on me that here was a man who had a sense of humour, a sexual identity, hopes and needs. I had seen the disability but had no awareness of the man.

My second key experience was at the same centre. A woman with cerebral palsy and mild learning disabilities came for a week's holiday. Her mobility was extremely limited, she had contracted limbs and uncontrolled spasms. Her speech was slow and difficult to understand. Laboriously, she communicated that she would like to go through our man-made pothole that consisted of a tunnel system in a confined space. I was game and sought assistance from a colleague. Between us we agreed that he would go at the front and pull, and I would take the rear and push. For me to go through the pothole took approximately 15 minutes. Three hours later we emerged battered, bruised and exhausted. The woman promptly began to cry and I feared we had physically hurt her. On asking what the matter was, she explained that everyone had said she was too disabled to come to an outdoor centre and she was wasting her time. Now, she said she was crying from happiness as she knew she could do anything she put her mind to. I was overwhelmed and realised that I could support people with disabilities to achieve their potential and that it was absolutely what I wanted to do. Incidentally, as a result of her experience at the centre, the woman went on to college and now lives independently with support from carers she employs.

Having discovered what I wanted to do, I looked for courses that would train me to work with people with disabilities. Nursing appeared to be the only course in which I could specialise from the start, so I applied. My family told me that nursing was a dead-end job with neither status nor money and that I would be unfulfilled and bored. Fortunately, I chose to ignore them and they have since admitted they were wrong. I learned from the woman at the centre that I too could achieve anything, if I was determined enough.

I began Project 2000 nurse training at Southampton University in 1994 and specialised in learning disabilities. Throughout the three years training I witnessed good and bad practice, learned the theory behind practice and learned about the type of nurse I wanted to be. One particular nurse stands out as being influential. She supervised me for a period of 18 months in a community team. Her outstanding feature was her honesty. She focused on the individual in a non-judgemental way but was always honest about the judgements that other people would make about individuals and the battles they would have to face. She always did what she believed to be right despite the pressures from services. This did not always make her the most popular practitioner but, at the end of the day, if she was able to go home and know that she had done her best for her clients, then she was happy.

I was not sure that I could ever be as tenacious as she was. However, I was determined that, if I were to undertake a piece of work, I would work with and listen to the individual. I also decided that I would give 100% effort, as anything less would be unacceptable.

When I completed my training, I would have liked to have taken up a post in the community. However, the NHS trust had no posts available. Therefore, I took a post in the private sector working with people with profound learning disabilities and epilepsy. All of the residents had complex health needs and severe physical disabilities. Initially, their level of disability scared me but I quickly learned how to deal with them and maximise their abilities. None of the 15 clients I cared for could speak, but they all communicated excellently if you were prepared to listen. Although I was ultimately in charge, and felt that responsibility acutely, I adopted a team approach. I believed that, because everyone felt valued and had a role, we had a productive and supportive staff team. Multi-tasking was a skill I quickly acquired and, whilst the 12 hour shifts were relentless and the job was both physically and emotionally demanding, I loved and was humbled by the clients and the people I worked with.

It was in this home that I began to develop my interest in epilepsy. I learned that epilepsy involved more than just medical issues: it touched on all aspects of a person's life, yet little attention was paid to anything other than the medication. Nursing seemed like the ideal profession to redress the balance. After a year in a residential setting, I returned to the NHS and the area I trained in by joining a community specialist health care team. Here, I undertook training in the field of epilepsy. Since this time, I have been supported to develop my practice at a local and national level, offering a specialist service to clients with learning disabilities, acting as an expert resource and developing services in the area.

Tristan's past

Tristan was a 21 year-old man with cerebral palsy and severe learning disabilities. At 14 he developed epilepsy and was referred to the neurology department of the local hospital where he was put on medication. In addition, he had syncope, which is a sudden drop in blood pressure that causes seizure-like episodes in which he lost consciousness and fell to the floor. Tristan lived at home with his family with regular weekend respite care. He attended a local day centre and enjoyed active pursuits such as walking and gardening. He was very active, had some stereotyped movements and verbalisations and shouted and screamed without provocation. He communicated non-verbally and it was difficult to establish his needs, as he did not use signing or symbol systems. When he was younger he used key words, but had not spoken for the past two years. No one could give a reason for this.

Because of the severity of his disability, Tristan relied on his mum for all his care. His dad worked during the day and had always taken more of a back seat in aspects of direct care, leaving his mum to be his advocate. This placed great pressure upon her and she felt isolated from society. Her life was destined to be different as a result of having a disabled child with chronic health needs. Research both in the field of learning disability and epilepsy has highlighted the impact on the quality of life of carers (Kendall *et al.*, 1999). This can often arise from feelings of loss that come from an expectation of what may have been and the ensuing guilt for wishing for something different (Morrey, 1995).

Although Tristan and his family often saw one of the community nurses, he was referred to me because of an increase in the number of his seizures. I was felt to be the appropriate person to take the referral because of the skills I had developed in the field of epilepsy. I saw the referral as a need for team working with his mum. I have undertaken additional training about epilepsy, which gives me additional knowledge and skills in the field, but Tristan's mum knew about her son; she lived with and managed his disability, and would continue to do so long after the case was closed to me.

I aimed to work with his mother to offer her support, knowledge and information and improve Tristan's seizures. I hoped, rather than presumed, that I could improve things for him and his family. Having knowledge about a medical condition that affected Tristan was not enough. I needed to find out what the family perceived his needs to be, and work with them to meet them in a way that they would find acceptable and achievable. This is supported by Witts (1992) who said that any intervention is unlikely to succeed unless it is rationally justified, there is a clear plan of action and all parties agree.

Carers state that the most valuable support they can be offered is someone who listens, with sensitivity and without judgement (Shanley & Starrs, 1994). The UKCC (1996) states that the nurse must 'act always in such a manner as to promote and safeguard the interests and well-being of patients and clients'. However, with a person with learning disabilities, who does not speak and has limited comprehension, this can be difficult to establish. Nurses often find themselves relying on information from those closest to the individual. In Tristan's case, this was his parents and, in particular, his mum. Although family carers will have the best interests of the individual in mind, nurses need to be aware that families will have had different experiences to the individual and will have different beliefs (Oliver, 1990). This can affect their views and the information they supply which, in turn, can affect the intervention. It is equally important for nurses to be aware of their own influences and the judgements they make and their potential effect on their decisions.

The initial visit

My first visit to the family was made with Tristan's community nurse who had built up a long-standing relationship with the family. We both felt it would be less intimidating if I was introduced. It was helpful to be able to observe their interactions, language, and level of formality and how they referred to shared events. This helped me to formulate a picture of how best to work with Tristan and his family, put them at ease and gain their trust, before establishing what they wanted from me.

I noticed that Tristan's mum had an informal relationship with the community nurse and seemed to gain comfort from a relaxed approach. Gathering information was interspersed with talk about the family, holidays and so on. The community nurse also offered information about herself that helped to make the relationship more equal. Clearly the relationship would take time to build, and a slow, informal approach seemed to be the most likely to succeed.

The issue presented to me was the increase in the number of Tristan's seizures. This was in line with the main aim of epilepsy care that is to 'achieve maximum health gain, reduce morbidity, and prevent avoidable mortality' (Epilepsy Task Force, 1998). Tristan's seizures had become more severe, with cluster seizures, which were difficult to bring under control. The increase in seizures presented an increased risk of death due to prolonged seizures (status epilepticus) and sudden unexplained death in epilepsy (Manford, 2002). Tristan was also at greater risk of sustaining an injury as he has tonic clonic seizures that cause a loss of consciousness and, invariably, a fall. Finally, the seizures were affecting his quality of life, as he was excluded from certain activities he enjoyed at his day centre because of the increased risk. Staff had assessed his activities and stopped those that were in the community and away from transport because, if an ambulance were required, it would need to have easy access.

I was happy to offer support but suggested that discussing the issues with their neurologist may be more appropriate, as he would be likely to alter the medication. Tristan's mum wasn't confident in neurology services and didn't feel she had a good relationship with Tristan's neurologist. It transpired that she often felt out of her depth with the medical terminology and, due to the time constraints, didn't feel she was listened to or able to ask questions. It helped that she felt able to offer this information at the first meeting as it allowed me a greater understanding of her emotional and information needs. The neurology department focused only on his epilepsy care, which conflicted with his mum's need for him to be seen as a whole person.

My initial interventions involved spending time with Tristan in a variety of settings, including his day centre, in his local community and within his home. His key worker and family were happy to facilitate this. Whilst he was unable to give me the verbal information I needed, I felt that, by spending time with him, I would become a face he recognised, which would be useful if I needed to support him to appointments. It also allowed me a degree of insight into his lifestyle and any difficulties that his family might face in caring for him and methods they had developed to manage his care. It helped his mum to believe that I cared about her son as a person and wasn't just assigned to work with his medical condition. Finally, I find it helpful to visualise a person when discussing them with others and it helps me to retain my individual focus.

An important discovery

I completed a detailed assessment of Tristan's epilepsy by using an individualised profile developed by a pharmaceutical company. This allowed me to gain a better understanding of his medical history, epilepsy and quality of life. It also gave me valuable time with his mum.

It is common for people with learning disabilities to develop epilepsy because the abnormal aetiology of the brain acts as a focal point for seizure activity (Betts, 1997). It is estimated that up to 50% of people with severe learning disabilities will have additional epilepsy that will often be difficult to diagnose and treat because additional health deficits can mask or interact with symptoms (National Society for Epilepsy, 1999).

It was necessary to be sure about the extent of Tristan's epilepsy. He had stereotyped movements and syncope attacks which could all be misdiagnosed and recorded as seizures, thus giving a false impression of the number of seizures he was experiencing. I checked with his mum that she recognised the different episodes and updated her knowledge using a comparison chart shown in Figure 12.1. (Hopkins *et al.*, 1995).

	Syncope	Seizure
Posture	Upright	Any posture
Pallor	Invariable	Uncommon
Onset	Gradual	Usually sudden
Injury	Rare	Not uncommon
Convulsions	Not common	Common
Incontinence	Unusual	Common
Unconciousness	Seconds	Minutes
Recovery	Rapid	Often slow
Post-ictal sleep	Rare	Common
Post-ictal confusion	Rare	Common
Precipitating factors	Crowds, lack of food, sudden pain or fright	Rare

Figure 12.1 Syncope and seizure comparison chart.

As I often find with parents of people with learning disabilities, Tristan's mum had never had his medical conditions explained to her. She said she had noticed a difference between Tristan's episodes but she was unaware that some were not caused by epilepsy. On further discussion I discovered that she had also experienced syncope throughout her teens and twenties. By clarifying the differences, we were able to accurately monitor the number of epileptic seizures using a seizure frequency chart, which I developed to encompass an accurate description of the event, possible triggers and the recovery period. Our discussion also helped in the identification of triggers which meant that Tristan could take steps to avoid any precipitating factors for either event.

I established that Tristan was having relatively few seizures, approximately eight a year, which is thought to be good seizure control in someone who has learning disabilities. Betts (1988) reported that the likelihood of achieving seizure freedom in someone with learning disabilities is less likely than in the general population. However, Tristan was having cluster seizures that were not being brought under control with the administration of rectal diazepam. This meant that the general practitioner needed to attend to give intravenous diazepam and Tristan was often admitted to hospital. This had a huge impact on the family, who were frightened by his seizures and felt inadequate at not being able to halt them. They were also inconvenienced by having to support him in hospital, as the ward staff didn't, or couldn't, adequately meet his needs, due to a lack of knowledge and resources (Welsh *et al.*, 2001). As a result, they feared the next episode and restricted his and their activities to ensure they were never far away from home. This meant that Tristan had to lead a restricted life and live with a medical condition that threatened his mortality.

By now I felt that I had to adopt a holistic approach to de-medicalise the condition, make her feel that I was interested in her son as a person, and acknowledge the impact epilepsy can have on a family. This was the first stage in breaking down barriers and building a relationship with the family.

Searching questions

The White Paper, *Valuing people* (Department of Health, 2001), stated that the role of the community nurse should be to facilitate access to generic services by people with learning disabilities. By compiling a detailed assessment of Tristan's epilepsy I had supported his access to neurological services by providing his family with information they would not have had time to collect in an outpatient's appointment. Taylor (1996) reported that these settings are not always conducive to good communication. I felt I had also begun to establish a good relationship with his mum that I hoped would help support the family in their visit to neurology.

I continued to visit the family in the run-up to Tristan's neurology appointment. His mum was clearly anxious about the change in seizure status and my visits gave her a chance to discuss her fears and ask questions in her own time and in the familiar environment of her own home. She asked repeatedly why it might have happened. Unfortunately, there was no definite answer to her question. Sometimes seizures change due to life experiences such as puberty or trauma (Sander, pers. comm.), but the reality is that there often is no obvious reason for the changes. Tristan's mum found this difficult to accept, and asked the question every time I spoke to her. I acknowledged that it was a hard fact to accept and that human nature required answers. I offered to give her some written information, which might answer her questions and confirm what I was saying and I suggested that she ring the helpline for the National Society for Epilepsy.

She refused the written information, saying she didn't like to read about 'it'. This was my first indication that she was having difficulties accepting the responsibility which was placed on her when she had a child with additional health needs and disability, possibly because she hadn't come to terms with the fact that her son would never live the life she had envisaged for him. However, she eventually rang the helpline, which confirmed what I had said. She then apologised for having done so. I reassured her that I had no problem with this and I was happy for her to seek information from as many sources as she felt appropriate. She began to relax with me and trust my knowledge.

I knew that adjusting Tristan's medication provided the best chance of improving his seizures and reducing his risks. However, for any proposed change to be effective, I knew that his mum, as the main care provider, would need to accept this. At this juncture, I felt that she was resistant to change because of her lack of understanding and faith in neurological services. At this point I realised that the majority of my work would be with his mum and that, despite the urgency, I would have to work at her pace. This left me with a dilemma. Tristan needed a medication review and was at increased risk whilst his seizures weren't being adequately treated. However, if his mum did not trust me or did not have enough information to make informed decisions on behalf of her son, then the chances of improving his epilepsy would be slim.

I began to build a better rapport with Tristan's mum from spending time with her and her son. This was important to me as I felt that the acceptance of her son's condition hinged on her feeling that she had support and someone whom she could trust and who wouldn't judge her. At this point she asked the searching question of why her son had been born disabled. The original referral was about Tristan's epilepsy, but I could not ignore her question without destroying the relationship we had built. Again I could not give her a firm answer, as it is often difficult to identify a specific cause of learning disability (Shanley & Starrs, 1994). She had debated the cause of his disability on a daily basis, wondering if she had done something to cause it during pregnancy. She was unable to discuss her fears with her husband and family and had lived with the guilt all her son's life. Her guilt was compounded; she believed her family had suffered as a result of having a disabled child. She had strong beliefs about looking after her family and felt that Tristan had demanded a large amount of her time and attention due to his needs.

It occurred to me that the lack of answers about the change in Tristan's seizure status mirrored the uncertainty about why he was born with a learning disability. I believed that if I was able to work with this long-standing issue then we would be able to tackle the epilepsy issues successfully. I set time aside to support her. I also suggested that she should see her general practitioner to discuss the issues. I was honest about my lack of skills in counselling and talked to her about the merits of seeing a professional but she said she trusted me and gained comfort from our meetings. I felt she had unresolved issues that were affecting her quality of life. I also suspected she was clinically depressed, as she spoke of feeling lethargic and disinterested and woke up early in the morning with a racing mind. She also looked physically tired and was making less effort with her appearance.

We discussed the possibility that she might be depressed and she agreed but refused to see her GP, as she was afraid he would prescribe her anti-depressants. When I asked why this would be a problem, she claimed she hated taking tablets. I wondered if this had any connection with her reluctance to adjust her son's medication. She seemed to believe that if everything had turned out as it should have, then there would be no need for anyone to have to take tablets, and doing so was an admittance of things being wrong. If she admitted things were wrong then she would have to face and deal with the painful reality and injustice of the situation.

Identifying the risks

Throughout our intense discussions about why her child had been born disabled, I tried to devote half of every session to discussing Tristan's epilepsy care, as the neurology appointment was looming ever closer. Tristan's mum was in a dilemma about whether to accept the epilepsy she knew or whether to try and improve it with another medication, which had potential side effects and no guarantees of working. I felt it was my duty to point out the risk to Tristan came from his increased seizures. People with epilepsy have a mortality rate that is three times greater than an individual without epilepsy (British Epilepsy Association, 1997). I was aware of the need to be sensitive but needed to make my point about the seriousness of letting the situation remain unchanged. I chose a day when she seemed more emotionally robust and allowed time either side to discuss any ensuing feelings. I was dreading discussing it. There is no good way to tell someone that their actions are putting another at risk of death. She was also vulnerable and I knew what I had to say would hurt and frighten her, yet I was able to empathise with her dilemma, as she could cause inadvertent harm to her son by changing his medication.

I was not looking forward to bringing up the issues of risk and the medication. I was aware of my body language, and adopted a relaxed and open posture so that Tristan's mum would feel that I was confident and willing to be questioned. I tentatively approached the subject, suggesting that the neurologist would want to change Tristan's medication because of the risks associated with his seizures. I was able to say this would be the case with certainty, as he was currently on the maximum dose of his anti-epileptic medication and only took one drug. I had also been meeting regularly with the neurology department as part of my role development as an epilepsy liaison nurse. This gave me insight into the way that it worked. Had I been unsure about what would happen during the appointment, I would have contacted Tristan's neurologist before speaking to his mum, so the information I gave her was a fact. I felt this was important, as she would have to deal with the uncertainty of whether any other medication would work, in what dose and whether there would be side effects. My aim was also to prepare her for the appointment so she could think about questions she might be asked and might want to ask, thus boosting her confidence and building a more positive relationship with her son's neurologist.

Tristan's mum surprised me by her insight into the risk factors. She also seemed comfortable to be discussing any changes with me in her own home, in her own time and in as much detail as she could deal with. This provided some reassurance for her, as she knew she would understand the process and rationale behind any proposals for change. She also knew that I would be monitoring Tristan with expert knowledge and, therefore, any problems would be picked up early. This made her an active participant rather than a passive recipient in her son's epilepsy care. Whilst this, in itself, brought responsibility, it also helped her to make informed choices and feel more in control.

As a result of my additional training in epilepsy, I was able to determine the medications that were likely to be used in Tristan's case as having better side effect profiles and being suitable for his seizure type. This meant I was able to discuss the drugs with Tristan's mum prior to the appointment so she was aware of their advantages and disadvantages. We then recapped on his seizures and compiled all the information the neurologist was likely to ask for. This succeeded in helping her to feel prepared for the appointment. Finally, I wrote to the neurologist outlining where I was in my work and the difficulties we were experiencing with Tristan's seizure control. My aim was that we should all focus on the same areas and use the limited time available to maximum advantage. This would leave more time for his mum to discuss any issues she had with the neurologist.

A key appointment

The day of the appointment arrived and I picked up Tristan and his mum. This simple act saved them a difficult bus journey, allowed me to run through the questions she wanted to ask, and gave extra physical support to Tristan, so his mum did not have to consider his needs instead of focusing on the appointment. We went into the appointment. I could tell by his mum's body language that she was inhibited but she was also prepared and rehearsed and this gave her the confidence to answer any questions. In turn, it gave a more accurate picture to the neurologist, and I was able to ensure that no important pieces of information were left out either because his mum didn't realise their importance or withheld information to avoid confronting her issues with medication changes. As a result, the neurologist gained an accurate snapshot of Tristan's epilepsy and the issues for him and his family.

As I predicted, the neurologist suggested adding in a second anti-epileptic medication. There was a variety of choices for Tristan's seizure types and his mum discussed the merits of each before a joint decision was made. I could tell that, for the first time, she felt as if she was part of the decision-making process and had contributed. This helped to improve her relationship with the neurologist and it boosted her confidence still further.

The neurologist and I devised a titration schedule to introduce the new medication and I ensured that Tristan's mum knew what side effects she was looking out for. My knowledge and experience was useful as people with learning disabilities are more susceptible to the effects of medication than the general population, so a cautious approach needs to be taken, with lower doses of the medication being given and a longer delay before the dose is increased (Shorvon, 2000). The new medication began the weekend before a bank holiday, so Tristan was not at the day centre and his mum could observe him. I rang on my return to work to see how the weekend had been and ensure that his mum felt supported during the changes. Fortunately, there were no problems and the medication could be titrated over a period of time.

A setback

I continued to support the family through this period and spent time observing Tristan. Sadly, after a few months, it became apparent that the new medication was having no effect on Tristan's seizures. Tristan was admitted into hospital three times within a period of six months. I accompanied him on one of these occasions and was shocked to see how ill he was. Despite having seen and dealt with many seizures, I had never seen a seizure that had such a profound effect on anyone. Tristan was unconscious for over an hour, despite the efforts of the medical team in the accident and emergency department. He had stopped convulsing but remained pale and unresponsive. It was difficult to believe that he could pull through at all, let alone without further brain damage.

It was not until then that I realised just how difficult it must have been for his parents. I understood that any change that could upset the status quo, such as a medication change, must have been an agonising decision to make. Whilst the aim is always to improve seizure control, there are no guarantees and there is even a risk of making the situation deteriorate. I realised how far Tristan's mum must have come in her thinking to even consider trying anything else. We now needed to revise his medication again, which meant looking at other drugs, with an increased likelihood of side effects. Understandably, Tristan's mum was not feeling very confident. It seemed to me that she had deteriorated emotionally with each seizure she witnessed and I needed to provide a lot of emotional support. I persisted in my quest to get her to seek professional support.

There was no point in keeping Tristan on a drug that was patently having no effect. We would also increase the likelihood of drug interactions if he were on poly therapy and so I discussed removing the additional medication and reintroducing another. Through lengthy discussions, his mum realised it was the only option if we were to try and improve his seizures. She was never going to feel happy about it, but she said she felt supported enough to go ahead. Because of my previous openness about the possibility of the medication not working, she still trusted the neurologist and me.

We scheduled another neurology appointment and I followed the same process after having tried it and found it to work. Once again we discussed the issues and another drug was introduced. At the same time the old drug was removed. It was made clear to Tristan's mum that each drug that failed left us with fewer options and decreased the likelihood of any drug being effective (Shorvon, 2000). I really felt for the family and desperately wanted to be able to give them some good news. However, I needed to be honest for ethical reasons and because it would destroy the trust I had built if I lied. I also needed to support them and tried to temper the facts with the hope that we still had drugs available. Also, I pointed out that more drugs were being developed as we spoke but, equally, there were no guarantees that the next one would work. Once again we devised a titration schedule, picked our start date carefully and began the new regime.

I don't think either of us had much confidence but I didn't let it show. Tristan's mum needed a lot of support, as she feared that removing a drug would cause his seizures to deteriorate, even though she knew the drug had had no effect on improving them. We went over the rationale and the action of the medications whilst changing the drugs. Because his seizures were infrequent, although serious, it was difficult to know if the medication was improving them. However, after several months with no seizures we were beginning to feel more confident. Tristan also began to improve in other ways: his mood was more stable and he regained communication skills thought to be lost, such as improved eye contact and the use of some words.

Looking to the future

As Tristan improved, so did his quality of life. The risks to him lessened, so activities he had previously enjoyed at day centre were reinstated with risk assessments that I helped to compile. Additional epilepsy training and supervision for staff helped them to regain their confidence and his mum to feel happier about this service. His mum improved emotionally and gradually began taking Tristan out further afield and on her own. She also spent more time with her husband, as she felt able to leave Tristan with others if they had training, which I provided. Finally, Tristan seemed to feel better. He had more energy and appeared to be enjoying life and getting more from it. To date, a year has passed and Tristan remains well with no further changes to his medication. I still see the family occasionally. There will always be neurology appointments and training needed for staff working with him, and there is always the possibility of his seizures changing again but, for now, we can relax, and Tristan and his family can get on with living their lives.

Reflections

I believe it is necessary to look at the whole picture when working with a client. The significant others in their life are often the key to supporting them. Whilst it is important to keep a focus on the task in hand, the direct route may not always be the best or most appropriate one to take. Much depends on the understanding and beliefs of the people you need to work with. People who are cared for formally or informally are reliant on their carers to varying degrees. Whilst there will be policies and directives governing formal care, no such guidance exists for families, which makes it essential to work alongside them and understand how being a carer impacts on them. It is also important not to underestimate how our own beliefs and influences affect the way we work with others.

Schon (1991) talks about two types of reflection: reflection in action, the process of simplistically examining what we do whilst we are doing it. The other, reflection on action, is the process of examining what we have done, how we feel the influences on our care and the consequences to our actions. This can be a formal process that takes place through supervision or it can be informal, and take place through thinking about what has been done and what we will do in the future to ensure the success of our intervention. Reflection is crucial to ensure best practice.

Formal knowledge allows us to practice within a given field and gives us the knowledge to be clear about our end goal and the interventions needed to get there. Informal knowledge supports us in knowing how to relate to people, understand what influences them and us, and build interpersonal relationships. It is essential to have both types of knowledge when delivering nursing care. With experience both our formal and informal knowledge grows and we become more experienced practitioners. However, reflection is an ongoing process, even in similar cases we work with individuals. One-size-fits-all intervention can never be as successful as an individual approach to care.

References

Barber, P. (1991) Caring: the nature of a therapeutic relationship. In: Perry, A. & Jolley, M. (1991) *Nursing: A Knowledge Base for Practice.* Edward Arnold, London.

Betts, T. (1997) *Epilepsy, psychiatry and learning difficulty.* Martin Dunitz, London.

British Epilepsy Association (1997) *Epilepsy Care: Making it Happen.* Epilepsy Advisory Board, London.

Department of Health (2001) *Valuing People: A New Strategy for Learning Disability for the 21st Century.* Department of Health, London.

Epilepsy Task Force (1998) *Service Development Kit.* Joint Epilepsy Council, London.

Kendall, S., Thompson, D. & Couldridge, L. (1999) *Investigating the Information Needs of Carers of Adults with Recently Diagnosed Epilepsy.* Buckingham Chilterns University College, UK.

Hopkins, A., Shorvon, S. & Cascino, F. (1995) Epilepsy. Chapman and Hall, London.

International League Against Epilepsy (1999) *Epilepsy '99: From Science to Patient.* Glaxo Wellcome, UK.

Manford, M. (2002) Convulsive Status Epilepticus. *Advanced Clinical Neurology Research,* **1**(6), 9–10.

Morrey, J. (1995) *Living with Grief and Mourning.* Manchester University Press, Manchester.

National Society for Epilepsy (1999) *Epilepsy: An Interactive Guide for Medical Professionals.* Parke Davis, London.

Oliver, M. (1990) *The Politics of Disablement: Critical Texts in Social Work and the Welfare State.* Macmillian Educational, Basingstoke.

Schon, D. (1991) *The Reflective Practitioner*. 2nd Edition. Jossey Bass, San Francisco.

Shanley, E. & Starrs, T. (1994) *Learning Disabilities: A Handbook of Care*. 2nd Edition. Churchill Livingstone, Edinburgh.

Shorvon, S. (2000) *Handbook of Epilepsy Treatment*. Blackwell Science, Oxford.

Taylor, M. (1996) *Managing Epilepsy in Primary Care*. Blackwell Science, Oxford.

United Kingdom Central Council (1996) *Guidelines for Professional Practice*. UKCC, London.

Welsh, R. & Wild, K. (2001) *Helping People with Learning Disabilities in Primary and Secondary Care*. West Hampshire NHS Trust, Southampton.

Witts, P. (1992) Patient advocacy in nursing. In: Soothill, K., Henry, C. & Kendrick, K. (1992) *Themes and Perspectives in Nursing*. Chapman Hall, London.

Chapter 13

Learning disability nursing: a model for practice

John Aldridge

Introduction

In the opening chapter of this book, John Turnbull describes how the background of learning disability nursing has led nurses to seek to differentiate their practice from that of other nurses, therapists and social workers. In Chapter 5, Gwen Moulster and John Turnbull explore how learning disability nurses work with individuals and their families and, in particular, what informs their thinking and decision-making. In Chapter 9, Jeanette Thompson and Sharon Pickering demonstrate the relevance of learning disability nursing to contemporary policy, philosophy and practice in the field of learning disability. Amidst these chapters an array of approaches used by nurses to promote the health, autonomy and, ultimately, the social inclusion of people with learning disabilities is described. This all adds up to a view of learning disability nursing as a dynamic and varied professional activity yet, paradoxically, one in which learning disability nurses still seek a more clearly articulated and coherent framework for practice. Given this, what follows in this chapter is an attempt to draw together some of the key issues for nursing practice in order to present a model for learning disability practice.

Nursing models in learning disability

The model that will be presented in this chapter is the *Ecology of Health Model*. This model developed out of the application in practice of the *Ordinary Living Model* for learning disability nurses that can be found in Aldridge (1987). Department of Health sponsored projects (Kay *et al.*, 1995), as well as research into learning disability nursing (Alaszewski *et al.*, 2001), have pointed to the need for nurses to be oriented towards the health of people with learning disabilities. However, before this can be accomplished there are several issues that still need to be satisfactorily defined and resolved.

First, what is meant by health in the context of learning disability? A biomedical model of health is too simplistic and has been criticised for focusing on people's impairments and contributing to a view of people with learning disabilities as dysfunctional and problematic (Wolfensberger, 1972). On the other hand, the social model of disability (Oliver, 1990) blames society for reacting negatively to a person's impairments but overlooks the effect that health can have on a person's quality of life (Gates, 1998). Therefore, it seems that a holistic model is required that explains the complex relationship between biological, psychological and social factors in health.

A second issue is what is the role of the learning disability nurse in providing holistic care to people with learning disabilities? Nursing has traditionally been oriented towards the physical and, to a lesser degree, psychological aspects of care. However, there is an incomplete understanding of the relationship between social activities and social processes in health. Therefore, there is a need for nurses to understand and to use social activities as a positive and intentional means of improving and maintaining health.

Third, how might nurses carry out a holistic assessment of the health of people with learning disabilities? Although a number of conceptual models provide an assessment framework it could be argued that none provide a satisfactory and complete understanding of the needs of people with learning disabilities. Although people with learning disabilities are people first, with the same needs as anyone else, they may also have a need for additional and specialised support that professionals and others should be able to identify in an accurate and reliable way. One approach to this might be to adapt existing nursing assessments or nursing models. However, there is a danger that a generic framework would fail to alert the assessor to important issues. Another problem is that any adaptation would destroy the coherence of the model and make it conceptually unsound. The best approach seems to lie in developing models that are based on a sound understanding of the dynamic nature of learning disability, its causes and influences, the context of care, and the aspirations of support services. The previous sentence deliberately used the plural, 'models', because this author believes that, such is the dynamic nature of care provision, professionals must have a range of conceptual models from which to select. The Ecology of Health Model is but one of these.

The Ecology of Health Model

The Ecology of Health Model can be seen in diagrammatic form in Figure 13.1 and should be referred to when reading the following description. The model was developed in response to practitioners' need for a model of nursing which specifically addresses the health care requirements of people with learning disabilities. In the context of this model, the *Person* may be seen as having physical and psychological elements which overlap to form the *Self* and which exist within a social environment. The social environment is not part of the Person but provides a supportive environment necessary to

Cognitive Processes
- Cognitive-developmental maturity
- Problem solving
- Learning, attention and consciousness
- Memory
- Moral reasoning
- Knowledge and understanding
- Effects of medication on cognitive processes

The Social Environment of Health
- Family membership, dynamics and processes
- Neighbourhood, housing, living conditions and circumstances
- Religion, culture and ethnicity
- Socio-economic status
- Formal and informal support networks
- Legal and policy issues

Affective Processes
- Emotional maturity
- Pleasure and gratification
- Motivation
- Mood
- Anxiety and confidence
- Giving and receiving affection
- Effects of medication on affective processes

Temporal Dimension
- The past
- The present
- The future

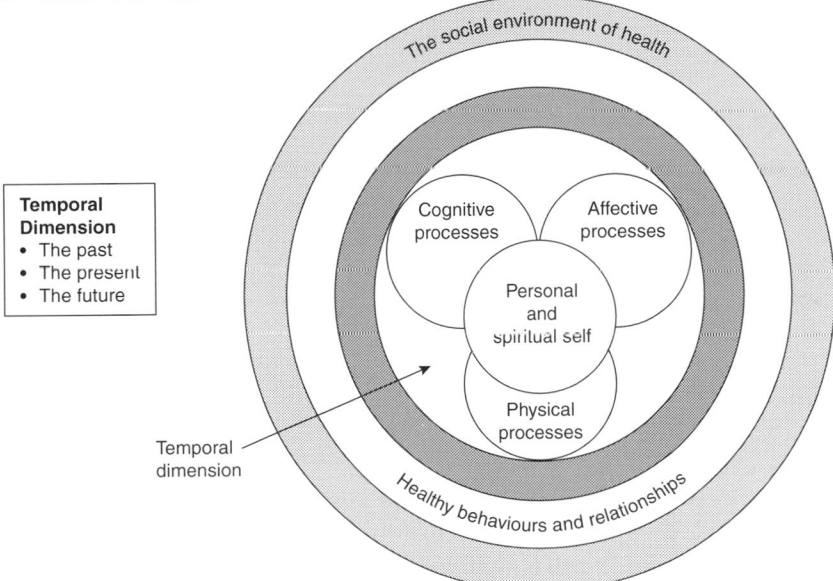

Physical Processes
- Physical growth and maturity
- Gastrointestinal system
- Musculoskeletal system
- Neurological system
- Endocrine system
- Body equilibrium systems
- Sensory systems
- Excretory systems
- Reproductive system
- Breathing system
- Circulatory system
- Skin and integumentary system
- Effects of medication on physical systems

Healthy Behaviours and Relationships
- Eating and drinking
- Moving and mobilising
- Maintaining personal hygiene
- Sleeping, resting and being comfortable
- Dressing and grooming
- Ensuring own and others' safety
- Perceiving and responding
- Knowing, learning and developing
- Making and maintaining relationships
- Expressing self and sexuality
- Communicating and self-determination
- Enjoying leisure
- Working and occupation
- Promoting health and well-being

Personal and Spiritual Self
- Language and self-expression
- Attachment, separation and loss
- Self-concept and self-perception
- Locus of control and self-empowerment
- Self-esteem and self-regard
- Religious, cultural and ethnic self
- Personal continuity and coherence

Figure 13.1   A representation of the Ecology of Health Model.

optimum physical and psychological functioning. The Person relates to their environment through interactive processes, termed *Healthy Behaviours and Relationships*. The dynamics and inter-relationships of these elements form an 'ecological' system – hence the name *Ecology of Health Model*.

The model was inspired by the work of Bronfenbrenner (1977, 1979), whose concepts of human development and interaction in an ecological framework provided the basis for an assessment and care planning approach which would encompass all of the possible elements which might contribute to an individual's health. It allows one to see the person and their world in their entirety and attempts to describe some of the interactions between those elements. This 'ecological' viewpoint informs the model's explanation of health, which may be defined as a dynamic and ever-changing state of individually defined optimal functioning and well-being, determined by the interplay between the individual's internal physiology and psychology and their external environment.

The model may be conceptualised as a three-dimensional figure representing the Person, surrounded in two dimensions by a number of concentric layers.

Layer 1

The Person is composed of four overlapping *domains*, collectively called *Personal Systems for Health*. This is seen as central for a number of reasons:

- It provides a person-centred perspective, from which we attempt to understand the individual's experience of the world, health and behaviour.
- Personal Systems for Health contain the core internal processes, the 'internal environment', which may contribute significantly to an individual's health.
- Personal Systems for Health contain four sub-domains, each of which may affect the others:
  - physical processes (or the physical self).
  - cognitive processes (the thinking and knowing self).
  - affective processes (the feeling self).
  - self-concept (literally the core of the individual, the essence of the person).

The model puts forward a view of humans as developing and growing individuals with a capacity to change and learn, irrespective of their chronological age. However, it also acknowledges that the rate at which people mature and change can be affected by specific difficulties. People with learning disabilities may be seen as having two kinds of interrelated impairments:

- Impaired physical or mental health, which may be acute, chronic or degenerative in its nature. The role of nursing in this context is to promote the individual's health, to ameliorate static or degenerative conditions, to prevent the deterioration of health and to provide palliative care if appropriate.

- Developmental impairments, which relate to physical, cognitive, emotional or self-concept elements. The role of the nurse in this context is to enable positive development, personal growth and independence.

The model further proposes that learning disability, especially where it is severe, may affect the individual in a number of ways that may differ from person to person:

- Physical impairments and physical health: damage to the brain and other bodily systems may result in frail physical health, a susceptibility to physical illness and disordered functioning of bodily systems, including the physical aspects of communication.
- Cognitive impairments: literally a learning disability, which may affect thought processes, the ability of the individual to know and understand the world or their ability to think and learn. Such an impairment may influence behaviour, interactions and, in some cases, mental health.
- Affective impairments: people who have learning disabilities may have difficulty in recognising, labelling, managing and expressing emotions. Their feelings may be the same as anyone else's but they may be expressed in unusual ways. They may express their feelings more openly, more strongly and with less inhibition. In some cases this might be labelled 'challenging behaviour'. An individual who has feelings that they have difficulty in managing and expressing may become distressed, dysfunctional or mentally ill.
- Self-concept may be affected by the above three elements and may be negative, positive or incomplete. We need to consider the degree to which the person knows himself or herself, both their physical and mental self, and the degree to which they feel happy and comfortable with themself. Self-concept develops and matures as we grow and develop. As adults we have a more complex and complete understanding of ourselves than we did as children. Self-esteem is affected by our life experience, but may also affect the ways in which we interact with others.

Layer 2

Surrounding the Person is a further domain, the *Social Environment of Health*, which represents the physical, political, social and cultural environment of the person. The social environment of health encloses all of the other domains; our personal lives, our behaviour and immediate relationships are played out within a number of *environments*:

- The *family environment*: people in our family and the relationships and interactions that we have with them.
- The *neighbourhood environment*: this includes the nature and quality of housing and neighbourhood, availability of local resources, accessibility and integration.
- The *cultural environment*: our religion and ethnic background may have considerable influence on our life patterns and beliefs and the readiness of others to accept us and value us.
- The *socio-economic environment*: this encompasses 'social class' (which might also be included in culture) and financial status. People who have learning disabilities are themselves likely to be relatively poor and, because of this, to have limited access to various activities and lifestyles.
- The *formal and informal supportive environment* includes the existence, or otherwise, of professional support systems, such as social workers or community nurses, and informal supports such as friends, self-help groups or neighbours.
- The *legal environment*: the influence and constraints of the law on individuals or groups.

Layer 3

Between the Person and the social environment of health lies the domain called *Healthy Behaviours and Relationships*, which represents the individual's relationships and interactions with all aspects of their environment and which acts as an interface between the internal and external environment. These may be listed as:

- Eating and drinking
- Moving and mobilising
- Maintaining personal hygiene
- Sleeping, resting and being comfortable
- Dressing and grooming
- Ensuring own and others' safety
- Perceiving and responding
- Knowing, learning and developing
- Making and maintaining relationships
- Expressing self and sexuality
- Communicating and self-determination
- Enjoying leisure
- Working and occupation
- Promoting health and well-being

Healthy Behaviours and Relationships is the meeting point between inner and environmental processes. These behaviours and relationships are supported by Personal Systems for Health, which enable the individual to carry out the activities that are listed under this heading. At the same time, the environments in which they take place influence the behaviours and relationships. In many ways, Healthy Behaviours and Relationships are the reason why we need good health. Health exists to enable us to do these things, to maintain our independence and to interact with our environment. If an individual has difficulty with eating and drinking, for instance, we need to consider why this might be. Is competence and independence in this activity affected by physical, cognitive or affective factors? What part does the environment have to play?

Layer 4

The third dimension, the *Temporal Dimension*, runs at right angles to all the preceding domains and represents the passage of time. It is composed of:

- *The past:* people, their health and behaviour do not exist in a vacuum; each has a history and a future, as well as a present. We often need to know how long situations and behaviours have existed and whether there are events that might be linked with this. It may be that the past contains secrets only known to the individual. In uncovering events, ideas or feelings we offer the possibility of dealing with them and offering therapy. The key issue here is the sensitivity with which we approach potentially difficult topics.
- *The present:* the present contains the situation as it is now; this may be the same or different to the situation in the immediate or distant past, and may be subject to change in the future. We may be able to discern patterns or themes emerging over time. The present contains actual health needs and health problems with which we have to deal now.
- *The future:* everyone has a future, although it may be brighter for some than for others. The future may be a source for optimism, something to look forward to, or it may be a source of dread, something to be avoided or fought against. For some individuals the future may represent more of the same, and this may involve more boredom, more abuse or more confusion. It may be that for some individuals the future is empty, they cannot predict what might happen and this in itself may be disturbing. A more optimistic view would be that nurses can help to influence the future in a positive way, to offer help, therapy and support. It is important that we make some attempt to look into the future, to think about the implications of past and present and to consider what options we might offer the individual and their family. The future contains potential health needs and health problems which we may be able to prevent or minimise, or we may need to be aware that those needs will require attention at some point.

Much of the inspiration for the Temporal Dimension is derived from *life story work* (Frost & Taylor, 1986; Ryan & Walker, 1993; Hussain & Racza, 1997) and this may provide a useful means of attempting both assessment and therapy. Although life story work has not been widely used in a therapeutic context in learning disability, its origins in fostering and adoption contain strong therapeutic elements and principles which may usefully be adopted when working with people who have learning disabilities and mental illness. Some useful discussion on the topic of working with sensitive issues is covered in Brigham (1998), McCarthy (1998) and Rolph (1998).

Each of the domains discussed above interacts with the others in a complex and dynamic manner. The relationships and interactions are not static, but develop over time. The interactions may take on a different form in different settings or circumstances or when different people are involved, and at different times each component of the domains will have a greater or lesser influence over the dynamic.

The role of the learning disability nurse within the model

The activities of nurses in supporting the health of individuals who have learning disabilities can be summarised under the following headings:

An assessment role
- Health surveillance, assessment and screening.

A teaching and developmental role
- Promotion of positive health and healthy behaviours.
- Promotion of personal growth, competence and development.

A therapeutic role
- Amelioration of static or degenerative conditions.
- Prevention of ill health or deterioration.
- Palliative care.

A healthcare role
- Planning, delivery and evaluation of healthcare programmes devised to meet individual health needs.
- Supervision of healthcare teams in the delivery of healthcare.

A networking and supportive role
- A supportive role in use of generic health services.
- Liaising with social care agencies to ensure positive social support.
- Supporting family carers to maintain the individual's positive health. Family-based work sometimes involves a decision about whether non-disabled family members' physical or psychological health needs are being met, but in such cases the use of a model which addresses those needs specifically is advocated.

Using the model

First principles

In order to understand how to use the Ecology of Health Model, the remainder of this chapter will set out some of the philosophical, organisational and practical issues when planning with people as well as explaining some of the terms that are associated with using the model. First of all, the model is underpinned by the need for plans to be:

- Person-centred
- Structured
- Purposeful.

As far as person-centredness is concerned, there is now a clear ethical and moral imperative that people with learning disabilities should be at the heart of any plans that are made for their lives. This applies equally to people with learning disabilities, who may be unable to communicate or to take part in any planning process, which makes it even more important that any conceptual model for practice should reflect person-centred principles. Although this imperative is clear and is supported by official guidance (Department of Health, 2001a), there still seems to be a fear that person-centred approaches represent a threat to professional practice (Turnbull, 2002).

A major question seems to be whether professional assessments and care plans reinforce a medicalised view of people with learning disabilities and how they fit in with life planning approaches. The Department of Health's guidance on this matter (Department of Health, 2001b) points out that person-centred approaches encompass a broad range of initiatives aimed at promoting the social inclusion of people with learning disabilities as well as their health and safety. The guidance is quick to point out that person-centred approaches should not replace other forms of assessment and care planning that are a necessary part of professional practice. As far as nurses are concerned, the Ecology of Health Model would allow them to make a structured and intelligent contribution to any life plans. The use of the model also promotes person centredness because it can be directly informed by contributions from the individual and has the capacity to reflect what is important and significant in an individual's life.

High quality care and support needs to be structured. There may be some people who feel that a too heavily structured approach to care devalues and objectifies people with learning disabilities. Research evidence and experience suggests otherwise. For example, many people with learning disabilities need specialist support that must be planned for and commissioned. This support would not be forthcoming without evidence that has been systematically collected. Furthermore, John O'Brien (1987) points out that his five accomplishments for people with learning disabilities can only be achieved through concerted action rather than being left to happen.

Finally, the process of assessment and care planning should be purposeful. This means that the individual and those caring for and supporting them should focus on what are the most valued outcomes for the individual. It is also important that these goals are clearly articulated and communicated.

Assessment

This discussion will now focus on the use of the Ecology of Health Model in practice. The full process is shown in diagrammatic form in Figure 13.2. From this diagram it can be seen that it is possible to use the model and to complete assessment in two ways.

(1) Completing a holistic assessment

The nurse must begin with the Personal Systems for Health, complete as much as possible and then move onto the Social Environment of Health, again completing as much as possible. Nurses will need to use their professional knowledge, experience and judgement regarding the importance of the elements for the person. It is unnecessary and undesirable to assess an element merely because it is listed as part of the model. The relevance of an element for the individual will depend on their stage in life, the nature of their disability, their social circumstances and the nature of presenting problems. The trigger points listed under each domain are merely a reminder of issues. They are neither prescriptive lists, nor are they exhaustive. Finally, the nurse must combine the observations from both of these domains to help in completing the Healthy Behaviours and Relationships.

By this stage the nurse should know quite a lot about the person and be able to form theories about *why* the person is able or unable to do certain things, or has difficulties in certain areas. Healthy Behaviours and Relationships do not need to be assessed separately from, and as well as, the other domains. The nurse draws information from what they have already discovered. It is more a matter of assembling the information into the form and structure that Healthy Behaviours and Relationships requires. The nurse must consider at all stages how the picture may have changed over time, what the present position is, and how it might change in the foreseeable future.

(2) Responding to a specific referral

Nurses may often receive a referral about a certain issue, which *should* fall into Healthy Behaviours and Relationships, but should certainly *not* relate to the Social Environment of Health. In this case a full holistic assessment is unnecessary because much time will be wasted on gathering irrelevant information and it is not what the referring agency or individual wants. The nurse should start with the referral area first and draw up as complete a picture as possible of what the individual is able to do, their behaviour and what constitutes the

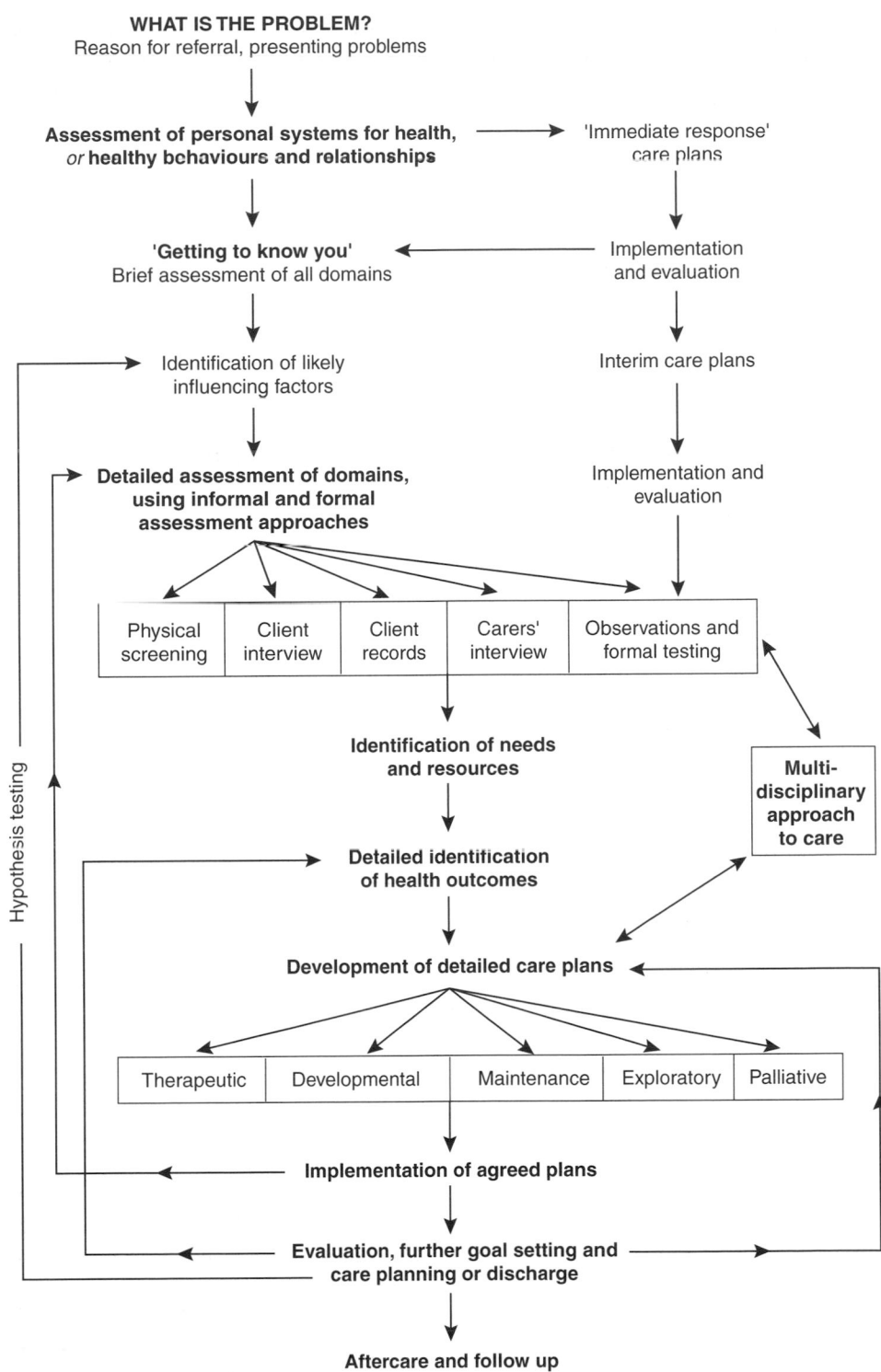

WHAT IS THE PROBLEM?
Reason for referral, presenting problems

Assessment of personal systems for health, ⟶ 'Immediate response'
or **healthy behaviours and relationships**　　　　care plans

'Getting to know you' ⟵ Implementation
Brief assessment of all domains　　and evaluation

Identification of likely　　　　Interim care plans
influencing factors

Detailed assessment of domains,　　Implementation and
using informal and formal　　　　evaluation
assessment approaches

| Physical screening | Client interview | Client records | Carers' interview | Observations and formal testing |

Identification of needs and resources

Multi-disciplinary approach to care

Detailed identification of health outcomes

Development of detailed care plans

| Therapeutic | Developmental | Maintenance | Exploratory | Palliative |

Implementation of agreed plans

Evaluation, further goal setting and care planning or discharge

Aftercare and follow up

Hypothesis testing

Figure 13.2　Care planning using the Ecology of Health Model.

problem. From this point the nurse would probably need to work backwards, by looking at Personal Systems for Health and the Social Environment of Health as a means of trying to find out explanations for the presenting problem. This should enable the nurse to see how to meet the person's needs and what should to be done to improve their health.

Care planning

As a health professional, the nurse needs to follow her assessment by describing outcomes for her interventions that are health oriented and which promote the person's health in some way. It is not always easy to think of *health* outcomes because the activities that people are engaged in are often seen as *social* actions. For example, people might regard leisure pursuits as primarily social activities. This would be a correct assumption but, from a health perspective, it is not the activity that is important so much as the outcome, which may include:

- Improved mobility through the use of physical activities.
- Relaxation through the use of calming and enjoyable activities.
- Improved perception skills through the use of activities involving looking and listening.
- Improved knowledge and understanding of money by calculating the costs and paying for activities or refreshments.
- Making and maintaining relationships by meeting new or old friends and sharing enjoyable activities and practising social skills.
- Self-expression through the use of dress and cosmetics.
- Enhanced self-esteem through the successful enjoyment of meaningful activities.
- Enhanced communication skills and self-determination through making choices about activities.
- Maintaining physical health through physical activity. Even going for a walk will generate aerobic activity, increase heart rate and may be used to aid weight reduction.

Therefore, the choice of leisure activity depends greatly on what needs to be achieved.

Care plans may fall into the following six broad categories:

(1) Therapeutic
(2) Developmental
(3) Exploratory/opportunity
(4) Palliative
(5) Maintenance
(6) Health promotion

(1)   Therapeutic

Care plans in this category are an attempt to improve the individual's health or functioning through a *therapeutic process*. The topic of therapeutic nursing has been discussed extensively elsewhere (McMahon & Pearson, 1998), but there is a need to differentiate here between a therapy and a treatment. It may be argued that most therapeutic approaches depend for their effectiveness on a relationship between the client and the person acting as the therapist, whereas a treatment can be carried out in an impersonal manner or even in the absence of a therapist (for example, medication).

As Gwen Moulster and John Turnbull describe in Chapter 5, the most powerful therapeutic tool that a nurse possesses is themselves, and it is often through the nurse–client relationship that a therapy is effective. If an individual is experiencing discomfort or distress, if their optimal health or functioning is compromised by a physical or psychological condition, then therapeutic approaches can be applied to alleviate or ameliorate the condition. These approaches may include:

- Physical therapies: the use of various forms of therapeutic touch, massage, manipulation, passive or active exercises, desensitisation.
- Psychological therapies: counselling, group and individual psychotherapeutic approaches, behavioural approaches, cognitive-behavioural and cognitive-emotive approaches, life story work.
- Combination therapies (those which have a physical and psychological element): relaxation approaches, t'ai chi, music and art therapies, any of the occupational therapies.

The outcome of any therapeutic care plan should be an increase in physical or mental health or well-being and a decrease in discomfort, distress or dysfunction.

(2)   Developmental

Developmental care plans are those intended to address the knowledge or skills of the individual through a process of teaching. Such teaching may use a behavioural, or precision skills teaching approach, or a more open 'learning by doing', or 'learning by experience' technique. Developmental care plans may be used to address the following issues:

- Social development: social skills, social behaviour and social interactions.
- Language development: the acquisition and improvement of vocabulary, language and paralanguage and communication skills (language and cognitive development are in many ways closely linked).
- Motor development: fine and gross motor skills, mobility and navigation.
- Sensory development: skills in using the senses; listening, looking and watching, attending.

- Cognitive development: the development of cognitive schemata to organise knowledge, categories (colour, size, shape, texture, temperature, foods, animals, etc.), strategies for memory and recall, morals and ethics (right and wrong), literacy and numeracy, cause and effect, practical problem-solving and so on.
- Self-concept development: body image, self-identity, self-esteem, self-expression.
- Self-care and independence: skills for everyday living (for example, eating and drinking, dressing, work and leisure skills).

(3) Exploratory/opportunity

These care plans might be used for discovering and exploring new ground with a relatively open outcome in mind. This is the only situation where a 'let's see what happens' approach might be condoned, though this needs to be carried out within reasonably controlled circumstances in order to minimise any unnecessary risk. Exploratory care plans might be used to give an individual an opportunity to experience something new in order to gauge their response. There should be a clear rationale for this, and a recognition of what the potential outcome might be. Additionally, this type of care plan might be used in order to find out more about the individual, especially if there is any doubt about the current state of knowledge; for instance, how much can the individual do for themselves, how much can they see or hear, to what extent are they able to use words relating to emotions? The reason that writing such a care plan has been advocated is that it gives us a structure, a purpose and a timescale, and the outcomes of such exploratory work can be evaluated.

(4) Palliative

This kind of care plan can be used in circumstances where the individual's health is static or deteriorating and where positive change through therapeutic work or treatment is undesirable or unattainable. The aim of such work would be to ameliorate or minimise any pain, discomfort or distress through the use of nursing intervention.

(5) Maintenance

These care plans are a way of making explicit the care issues which need specifically attending to but in which the motive is to maintain, rather than change, the client's status. Maintenance care plans are essentially supportive in their nature (Levine, 1977), but may be necessary in cases where prevention of deterioration requires care to be defined in detail.

(6)   Health promotion

Health promotion care plans might be used when there is a wish to initiate change in the client's health status. Here, it should be remembered that health promotion is a proactive process and healthcare is a reactive process. Health promotion care plans are essentially preventive in nature because they seek to address the underlying causes of potential health problems and to interrupt ill health. For instance, pressure sores might be prevented by addressing the causative factors such as body build, diet and seating.

Implementation

Implementation of care plans can seem to be a simple case of doing what is planned. On one level this is quite true but, as the following discussion points out, there are a number of factors that the nurse must be aware of.

First, implementation of care plans can be conceptualised as:

- Effective, if its outcomes are met. This is the aim that should be achievable if resources are well mobilised.
- Ineffective, if its outcomes are not met. This is perhaps acceptable if the nurse and the team are doing their best within the resources that they have available.
- Inappropriate or counterproductive, if it is not carried out properly. This is inexcusable in any circumstances and is a genuine failure to deliver the care to which clients have a right.

Effective implementation clearly has two associated elements:

- Proper implementation of planned action: did the care team *really* do what they should?
- Accurate recording of actions and outcomes of actions: what did they do, when, what happened as a result?

Any nurse who writes a care plan is only one of a number of cogs in the machine. Nurses are members of a care team that exists to work together in order to deliver care to the client. Nurses rely on other members of the team to carry out care plans properly, skilfully and fully, when they are not there. If this is to happen, a number of factors need to be in place:

- A care team whose members *all* understand the care plan.
- A care team with the skills to carry out any interventions or actions involved.
- A care team who *all* need to 'own' (in an emotional sense) the care plan, to believe in its purpose and effectiveness.
- Appropriate help and support to do the job properly.
- The team's implementation *must* ensure continuity of approach and effort.

A care plan can only be evaluated properly if there is an accurate record of its implementation. Again, recording is a team effort, and the nurse has to rely on others to record what happens when he or she is not present. The factors necessary for good recording are:

- Clear and easy to use systems for recording that are understandable and that do not require large amounts of time and effort to complete.
- A 'foolproof' system that clearly indicates if it is not fully completed.
- A system that gives accurate and complete data and that is easy to analyse at the time of evaluation.
- A care team whose members are *all* motivated to record implementation fully and accurately and who know how to use the system.

Implementation of care plans is clearly about team work. Indeed, good care plans may founder simply because they have not been properly implemented by all members of the team. Effective implementation needs the following skills:

- Skills of care planning in such a way that involves the individual, where possible and all of the team at all levels, usually through group decision-making in care planning meetings and reviews.
- The nurse may need skills in 'selling' the care plan to the team.
- Good practice skills. The nurse needs to be innovative and proactive and open to developing skills through education and reflective practice.
- Good teaching skills. Other people, including the individual, may need to be shown how to do something differently.
- Good recording skills. Develop systems of recording that are user-friendly, accurate and readily available. The individual and members of the team may need to be taught how to complete recording sheets properly.
- Motivation skills. If the plan is not going well, how does the nurse maintain motivation as well as that of others? This can partly be answered by the skill of setting outcomes that are easily achievable, using errorless learning approaches and by celebrating achievements with the client and the care team.

Evaluation

Evaluation provides an opportunity for everyone involved in implementing the plan to test out the hypotheses regarding cause and effect in the client's life and the effectiveness of any planned interventions. If recordings have been accurately and consistently made, there should be sound data upon which to base any judgements about future action. If there is confidence in the data and objectives have been attained, then there is an obvious reason to celebrate. If objectives have not been achieved, then this may be for a number of reasons that could be used to inform future plans. For example:

- Was it something about the client?
  - How well motivated were they?
  - How might the client's motivation be optimised?
- Was it something about the circumstances?
  - Were there any coincidental changes in medication, living circumstances, day services, other peoples' behaviour that could have affected the implementation of the plan?
  - How might the impact of these factors be minimised in the future?
- Was it something about the way that the care plan was written?
  - Was the outcome too difficult to achieve in the circumstances, given current resources and the powers of the client?
  - How could the outcome or method be changed to make it more achievable?
- Was it something about the implementation of the care plan?
  - Did *all* the members of the care team carry it out properly?
  - Did *all* the team members carry it out at all?
  - Did the team have the skills to carry out the plan?
  - How could continuity be achieved?

Evaluation can also be seen as part of an assessment process. By implementing care plans, whether successful or not, everyone will have learned a great deal about the client, which can be added to the assessment.

'Closing', aftercare and follow-up

Following the closure of long-stay hospitals and other long-term health service facilities, nurses and other health professionals have had to confront the issue of discharge and what this might represent in terms of their practice with people with learning disabilities. This issue undoubtedly needs further debate. However, there is a case for proposing that health services for people who have learning disabilities need to move towards a model of assessment and intervention in which there is an overt objective of eventual discharge, or 'closure' once the circumstances are right. In such a model, there will be some individuals who only need specialist health services temporarily and who move through the service relatively quickly. At the same time, there are likely to be a number of individuals whose progress is very slow. For these individuals, it may be that closure is aimed for but never actually achieved within their lifetime.

At the point of discharge, or closure, the nurse and the team need to consider the following points:

How can the health improvements be consolidated for an individual?
- What are the wishes of the client, their family or carers?
- Do the carers need to be educated or informed?
- Does the client need to be educated or informed?

- What changes to the individual's lifestyle should be proposed?
- What is the nature of the environment and circumstances into which the client will be discharged?

What aftercare and follow-up procedures need to be implemented?
- How might the individual's health be maintained?
- Who is the most appropriate person to carry out the aftercare?
- What does the person need to do in order to ensure the greatest long-term effect of the period of healthcare?
- Is there a need for continuing domiciliary healthcare?
- Is there a need for periodic readmission, re-referral or 'top up' of a programme?

Conclusion

It has only been possible within one chapter to present an outline of the Ecology of Health Model and how it can be used. It is also important to recognise that the model is a tool to be adapted (within reason) and should not be followed slavishly or rigidly. However, there are a number of key features and principles related to the model that are worthwhile reiterating.

Planning effectively with and for people with learning disabilities should be a logical and objective process designed to optimise the individual's progress toward health goals. Such a solution-focused and goal-directed process is the only ethically defensible approach, but it does require the additional structure of a nursing model to help with the task of assessment and care planning. The Ecology of Health Model is one such model of nursing that has been designed to be applicable to the full range of learning disabilities. It is also a model that acknowledges the significance of social factors in the person's life and the current context of care provision that distinguishes between health and social care.

References

Alaszewski, A., Gates, B., Motherby, E., Manthorpe, J. & Ayer, S. (2001) *Educational Preparation for Learning Disability Nursing: Outcome Evaluation of the Contribution of Learning Disability Nurses within the Multi-professional, Multi-agency Team.* English National Board, London.

Aldridge, J. (1987) Initiating the use of a nursing model: the importance of systematic care planning – a ward clinician's perspective. In: Barber, P. (ed) *Mental Handicap: Facilitating Holistic Care.* Hodder & Stoughton, London.

Brigham, L. (1998) Representing the lives of women with learning difficulties: ethical dilemmas in the research process. *British Journal of Learning Disability*, 28, 146–50.

Bronfenbrenner, U. (1977) Towards an experimental ecology of human development. *American Psychologist*, 32, 513–31.

Bronfenbrenner, U. (1979) *The Ecology of Human Development: Experiments by Nature and Design*. Harvard University Press, Cambridge, Mass.

Department of Health (2001a) *Valuing People: A Strategy for Learning Disability for the 21st Century*. Department of Health, London.

Department of Health (2001b) *Towards Person-centred Approaches: Planning with People. Guidance for Implementation Groups*. Department of Health, London.

Frost, D. & Taylor, K. (1986) This is my life. *Community Care*, 7th August, 28–9.

Gates, B. (1998) New health agenda for learning disabled people: reflections on platitudes and rhetoric. *Journal of Learning Disabilities for Nursing, Health and Social Care*, **2**(1), 1–2.

Hussain, F. & Racza, R. (1997) Life story work for people with learning disabilities. *British Journal of Learning Disability*, **25**, 73-6.

Kay, B., Rose, S. & Turnbull, J. (1995) *Continuing the Commitment: The Report from the Learning Disability Nursing Project*. Department of Health, London.

Levine, M. (1977) Nursing ethics and the ethical nurse. *American Journal of Nursing*, May edition, 845–9.

McCarthy, M. (1998) Interviewing people with learning disabilities about sensitive topics: a discussion of ethical issues. *British Journal of Learning Disability*, **26**, 140–45.

McMahan, R. & Pearson, A. (eds) (1998) *Nursing as Therapy, 2nd edition*. Stanley Thornes, Cheltenham.

O'Brien, J. (1987) A guide to personal futures planning. In: Bellamy, C.T. & Wilcox, B. (eds) *A Comprehensive Guide to the Activities Catalogue: An Alternative Curriculum for Youth and Adults with Severe Disabilities*. Paul Brookes, Baltimore.

Oliver, M. (1990) *The Politics of Disability*. MacMillan, Basingstoke.

Rolph, S. (1998) Ethical dilemmas in historical research with people with learning difficulties. *British Journal of Learning Disability*, **26**, 135–9.

Ryan, T. & Walker, T. (1993) *Life Story Work*. British Agencies for Adoption and Fostering, London.

Turnbull, J. (2002) Editorial: careless talk. *Learning Disability Practice*, **5**(2), 2.

Wolfensberger, W. (1972) *The Principle of Normalisation in Human Services*. NIMH, Toronto.

Chapter 14

Sustaining learning disability nursing practice

John Turnbull

Introduction

The opening chapter outlines the key aims of this book, which are to explore the experience of being a learning disability nurse and to deepen readers' understanding of what learning disability nurses set out to achieve and what they draw upon to inform their practice. It is hoped that the nine practice-based chapters and the four reflective and theoretical accounts have combined to uncover the richness and complexity of nursing practice.

Following on from this, the aim of this concluding chapter is to pose an important question, which is 'how will the skilled and accomplished practice of the learning disability nurse be sustained into the future?' At face value, it could be supposed that this question makes two assumptions: first, that the continuation of the learning disability nurse will remain a strategic priority for policy makers in nursing and the field of learning disability and, second, that learning disability nursing will continue in its present form. Given the history of learning disability nursing, some would say that these are optimistic assumptions to make. Clearly, it would be impossible to predict with any certainty at what point in the future or under what circumstances changes might occur. On the other hand, it would be naïve to assume that there will be no change. Therefore, this chapter will explore what is required to sustain learning disability nursing practice, whilst alluding to possible threats to the profession or factors that might inhibit nurses from practising at their best.

Recruiting to the profession

Any investigation into the future of learning disability nursing practice must start by posing the question of how recruitment to the profession might be affected by current trends. Recent years have witnessed considerable activity within nursing to solve a recruitment crisis that was caused by a combination of factors, including an ageing workforce, poor retention, an increase in the demand for nursing skills and an increase in alternative employment opportunities. It is unclear whether these conditions have been replicated within learning disability nursing, though previous experience suggests that recruitment patterns for learning disability nurses are different to their colleagues in other branches. For example, it was once assumed that the families living in the staff accommodation that was built within the grounds of the long-stay learning disability hospitals would provide a steady supply of recruits to nursing posts and that the demise of those hospitals would trigger a recruitment crisis. It is a fact that alarm over a decline in the number of students entering learning disability nurse education (Nursing Times, 1991) led the English National Board to call on the Department of Health to take action. However, the reasons for this decline probably had more to do with uncertainty about the role of the learning disability nurse in the community than the dispersal of staff accommodation. This is perhaps indicated by the upturn in recruits during the past decade now that the role of the learning disability nurse is more established.

It is also worthwhile recalling the reasons for entering the profession given by the authors of the practice chapters in this book. Although they are not a representative group, they describe a desire to help people with learning disabilities access their rights, to help them become more independent and enjoy a better quality of life, to do something worthwhile and make a difference. In almost all of their accounts, these feelings were triggered by encounters with people with learning disabilities, many of which were accidental meetings.

The issue of what motivates people to become learning disability nurses is an important, yet under-investigated, area and it is therefore hazardous to make any firm predictions about whether the public's interest in learning disability nursing as a career will be sustained. A factor that could potentially affect motivation would be a change in the public's perception of the needs of people with learning disabilities. For example, if as a result of social policy people are more visible and are afforded equal status by the public, then this may not arouse such a strong desire to right any perceived social injustice. While this must be considered a possibility, the pace of social change might make it a fairly distant prospect. Therefore, it could be hypothesised that the reasons for wanting to work with people with learning disabilities are likely to survive any short- to medium-term social and economic trends. In fact, as some of the contributors reported that a chance encounter with a person with learning disabilities was a factor in them seeking nurse training, social trends might actually increase opportunities for this to happen. For example, the segregation of up to 60 000 people with learning disabilities in long-stay hospitals in the past (Race, 1995) was mirrored by policies of segregation in employment and education during much of the 20th century. The closure of hospitals and the introduction of policies and legislation that have been driven by goals of greater social inclusion may have resulted in greater opportunities for members of the public to interact with people with learning disabilities.

Although members of the public may still want to become learning disability nurses for the same reasons as before, a key issue is whether there will continue to be opportunities for them to do so. As with other professions and occupations, learning disability nursing will be affected by changes in the job market. This is a complex area and it is virtually impossible to make firm predictions about what might happen to learning disability nursing in this context. However, it is more likely that opportunities will be affected by changes in nurse education itself. This raises the thorny issue of the future of the branch programme in learning disability. This is an issue that has been debated at great length before, and there is no desire here to resurrect all of the arguments about the advantages and disadvantages of change. Instead, the rest of this section will rehearse some of the possible changes to the branch programme and explore their implications for future recruitment of learning disability nurses.

Whatever the future of nurse education, as far as learning disability nursing is concerned the scenarios fall into three different categories:

- *The removal of the specialism:* this scenario would see learning disability nursing removed completely from nurse education at pre- and post-qualification levels.
- *The postponement of the specialism:* this scenario can be further divided into two parts. The first would see learning disability specialist education removed from pre-registration education but replaced by a post-registration qualification. The second variation on this would occur if a foundation course in health care or nursing gave a nurse a 'licence to practice'. This nurse could then acquire academic credits and specialise in aspects of learning disability practice. This scenario would fit with current proposals contained within the report *Agenda for Change* (Department of Health, 2003).
- *The retention of the specialism:* there would be a specialist programme, possibly akin to the current one, along with a separate award that could be registered with the Nursing and Midwifery Council.

The *removal of the specialism* scenario would result in decisions needing to be taken about the future provision of an award in learning disability. This could take the form of a national vocational qualification pathway, possibly extending the current learning disability awards framework (Department of Health, 2001). Given the fact that many learning disability nurses have a greater affiliation to the client group rather than the profession, it might be supposed that this scenario would not affect recruitment. In fact, this could assist recruitment because there may be members of the public who are currently put off from applying for nurse education courses because of its association with a medical, and discredited, model of care and support.

The first version of the *postponement of the specialism* scenario is one that has already received attention because it was the option that the panel of experts chose at the Consensus Conference on the future of learning disability nurse education in 1993 (Brown, 1994). Despite being chosen by the panel, as Norman *et al.* (1996) pointed out, this option received considerable criticism from the profession. As far as recruitment is concerned, the postponement of the specialism would have a devastating effect because it is highly unlikely that nurses would want to undergo up to three years of generic nurse education in preparation for studying and practising in the field of learning disability. Because the second version requires the nurse to complete a foundation course, its impact on recruitment into a learning disability nursing specialism would crucially depend upon the length of this course and whether its content would offer opportunities to work with people with learning disabilities. In other words, if the foundation course is lengthy, for example two years, and has no learning disability content, then it is unlikely to recruit students to learing disability nursing.

In the final *retention* scenario, it is assumed that a specialist programme for learning disability nursing is retained, but this does not necessarily mean that it would take the form of the current nurse education system. Whatever the shape of this course, people might be attracted to it in the same numbers as before, as long as the qualification retained its currency in health as well as social care.

Converting values into action

Moving on from the issue of recruitment, the remainder of this chapter will explore topics that have been raised through research into learning disability nursing, and other key documents that are regarded as significant to how nurses will practice in the future. The first of these topics concerns how the values and principles that underpin learning disability nursing practice could be successfully translated into action in the organisations in which nurses work. Learning disability nurses have consistently reported how important it is in sustaining their motivation that the people who they support become more independent and are included in the communities in which they live (Clifton *et al.*, 1992; Norman *et al.*, 1996). Obviously, learning disability nurses are not unique in wanting this, and now, with others from the field of learning disability, they want to promote the values of rights, choice and inclusion that are set out in the *Valuing People* White Paper (Department of Health, 2001). In the future, a key issue would be how these values could be increasingly brought in to learning disability nurses' practice.

Although precise figure are difficult to obtain, it is safe to assume that the majority of learning disability nurses work within National Health Service Trusts. Whereas there were once fourteen NHS Trusts that focused exclusively on services for people with learning disabilities, there are currently only three. Most learning disability services are now delivered within combined mental health and learning disability NHS Trusts, and some are delivered from within the newer Primary Care Trusts. The remainder of learning disability nurses are employed by independent sector social care or health providers, while others work for Social Services Departments. Although it is extremely early to tell, a preliminary assessment of how Learning Disability Partnership Boards are implementing targets set out in *Valuing People* suggests that those proposals have made little or no impression on the culture of services (MENCAP, 2003). Explanations for this are not straightforward. However, at an organisational level, it is possible that many NHS Trusts and Social Services Departments have such diverse functions that they find it difficult to translate the values within the learning disability community into action. This is in spite of the recent emphasis on the need for person-centred practices across the range of health services and the fact that many NHS Trusts and Social Services Departments clearly espouse a humanistic vision as part of their aims and objectives. Proctor's analysis (2000) suggests that many areas of the health service set out to improve the health of local populations but, in practice, the staff who work in them translate this into curing illnesses within the community and trying to restore individuals to better health. This is in contrast to the health care aims of learning disability nursing which views health care more as a collective and political activity that can empower people by opening up life choices and by removing sources of disability. These differences can manifest themselves in the way that managers behave, what gets measured within organisations and, ultimately, what is seen as a successful service. If this results in learning disability nurses and their colleagues within multi-functional organisations receiving less attention, this will inevitably perpetuate misunderstanding of the value of nursing in this field and will not sustain good quality practice. This trend was also detected by Alderwick (1998) and her colleagues who surveyed forty-one professional heads of nursing, psychology and occupational therapy in learning disability services in a range of NHS Trusts in the UK. The survey asked whether services in the Trusts were based on clear values. Although professional heads in all types of Trust responded affirmatively to this, two-thirds of respondents in mixed Trusts replied that their mission statement could be improved, compared to 84% of respondents in the single speciality learning disability Trusts. A further question asked how readily the learning disability services could determine its own strategic direction. Disappointingly, only half the respondents in mixed Trusts replied 'extremely well' or 'pretty well' to this question, compared to well over 80% in the single speciality Trusts.

In the face of evidence such as this, it would be wrong to believe that only single specialty learning disability organisations in health and social care will provide the answer for the future of learning disability nursing. There may be benefits to learning disability nurses of being in a mixed organisation, such as extra resources for further training or access to research and development opportunities. However, that means that steps need to be taken at an organisational, collective and individual level to ensure that values are implemented. Iles (2003) proposes that organisations that are flexible, that value creativity and that adopt a flat structure are more likely to promote person-centredness. Likewise, Turnbull (2002) suggests that values-led organisations are those that encourage staff to think for themselves and listen which, in turn, enhances their capacity to problem solve and innovate. Proctor (2000) and James (1994) add to this by suggesting that health service managers can become frequently dislocated from the process of caring and supporting clients and service users. When this happens, managers are tempted by short-term, expensive, technological solutions to achieving their aims. This is probably more likely to happen in the current climate of targets and policy imperatives. Proctor and James both propose that health care aims can be achieved more satisfactorily and accountability strengthened when managers are informed about the consequences of their decisions, by creating opportunities for the public and managers to meet each other. Whereas this is more likely to happen at a senior level in single speciality organisations, people with learning disabilities may not get the opportunity to meet with senior management in mixed organisations. Therefore, nurses and their colleagues need to find ways of making this a priority for the Trusts in which they work.

At a collective level, nurses can be helped in a range of ways to put their values into practice. In recent years, one of the main forms of collective action has been the rise in the popularity of networking, where nurses and others from different organisations come together to learn from each other and support each other's practice. The National Network for Learning Disability Nurses is perhaps the most prominent of networks and further information can be found at the Foundation of Nursing Studies' website. Stewart and Todd (2001) explored the roles of community learning disability nurses who reported that networking was an important component in maintaining their confidence. The Welsh Assembly Government's (2002) consideration of future roles for learning disability nurses recognised that the isolation of learning disability nurses could pose a barrier to good practice, and therefore recommended more networking between nurses. Likewise, a recent Scottish Health Service (NHS Scotland, 2002) document on the nursing contribution to the lives of people with learning disabilities proposed that nurses should come together in networks to counteract the effects of isolation.

On an individual level, reflective practices such as clinical supervision are widely thought to bring benefits for service users and nurses themselves by enabling nurses to refocus their practice in order to retain their person-centred aims and goals (Wolverson, 2000; Bending, 2001). For example, in Blackmore's (2001) small-scale study of learning disability nurses' experiences of advocacy, respondents reported that clinical supervision helped nurses to re-connect with their values and recognise the role of advocacy in supporting people with learning disabilities. The Welsh Assembly Government's document on learning disability nursing also promoted clinical supervision as a means of nurses and managers monitoring the move towards more person-centred services.

Although it is safe to assume that the use of clinical supervision within nursing is becoming more widespread, it remains to be established just how successfully it is applied within learning disability nursing. As it was pointed out in the opening chapter of this book, many learning disability nurses will find themselves working in social care settings where they may feel unable to access an appropriate clinical supervisor, and they may need to make a special effort to do so under these circumstances. Of course, whether the nurse and their supervisor would be able to conduct their sessions during working hours is questionable.

Lifelong learning

Clinical supervision is one of the key mechanisms through which nurses maintain their professional skills and standards, and this is commonly called *continuing professional development* (CPD). CPD is also a central feature of the Government's pursuit of a culture of lifelong learning in the National Health Service (Department of Health, 1997). It enables nurses to keep up with developments in their field but it also equips them for current and emerging specialist areas of practice. Under the proposed arrangements for the future pay system in the National Health Service (Department of Health, 2003), professional development will also be important as it is the Government's intention to link the development of extra skills and responsibility with pay.

As far as specialist practice is concerned, research has demonstrated that many learning disability nurses are fulfilling specialist roles in areas such as challenging behaviour, mental health, epilepsy and profound learning disability (Clifton *et al.*, 1992; Alaszewski *et al.*, 2001). Demographic and strategic change also means that learning disability nurses should look towards developing new specialisms. For example, people with learning disabilities are living longer and their life expectancy now approximates that of the general population (Hogg *et al.*, 2000). As a consequence, people with learning disabilities will become susceptible to diseases and illnesses of old age, such as dementia and cancer. As Northfield and Turnbull (2001) discovered, comparatively little is known about how to support a person with learning disabilities who has cancer and there could be a need for nurses to develop specialist knowledge in this area, especially to co-ordinate the support of different services. There may also be a need for specialist support for people with Down's syndrome who develop Alzheimer's disease and, as people with more profound learning disabilities survive beyond infancy, there are other similar challenges. Strategic changes, such as the introduction of health facilitation (Department of Health, 2001) will mean that learning disability nurses are likely to develop expertise in this area.

The key issue for learning disability nurses is how specialist practice can be supported and sustained. On a positive note, the Department of Health has announced that £100 million will be set aside over the next three years to support nurses who are developing their skills and taking on extra responsibility in order to meet the requirements of *Agenda for Change* (Nursing Times, 2003). This will be welcomed but learning disability nurses and their leaders will need to be vigilant about how this money is allocated so as not to repeat mistakes of the past. For example, taking on new roles and maintaining specialist practice will require significant input from higher education, as well as more senior managers and nurses in the practice environment to provide mentoring and placement opportunities. As Parahoo and Barr's (1994) survey of community nursing illustrated, this practice has not always been supported and accredited by higher education institutions. This is not to say that nursing practice has been poor. On the contrary, as Turnbull (2000) stated, learning disability nurses have been practising to a very high standard. However, they have been poorly served by the higher education system, primarily because small numbers of specialist staff have meant that education programmes are seen as unviable. The competitive environment between universities that is perpetuated by workforce confederations and, in the past, by education consortia in England, has discouraged universities from collaborating to develop ways of accrediting specialist practice. On the other hand, it must be acknowledged that learning disability nurses can sometimes ignore or underplay the significance of education programmes because they do not specifically mention learning disability nurses or because they are designed primarily for other branches. These problems must be solved if practice is to be developed and accredited. The National Nursing Review in Scotland (NHS Scotland, 2002) acknowledged this problem and strongly recommended that post-registration education is implemented to improve to help nurses better fulfil their roles. However, avenues are opening up in the areas of e-learning and open learning that could provide other ways of supporting learning disability nurses.

Leadership and management in learning disability nursing

Closely related to discussion of future specialist roles and lifelong learning is how the context of service provision will support leadership and management in learning disability nursing. Research has consistently demonstrated support from senior managers, professional colleagues and carers for learning disability nurses to take up co-ordinating and management roles. In particular, in Stewart and Todd's (2001) research, professional colleagues saw nurses occupying 'gatekeeping' roles in the future. This could be translated to mean care management or health facilitation, a role recommended for nurses by the *Valuing People* White Paper (Department of Health, 2001). Norman *et al'*.s (1996) investigation of learning disability nursing roles supports nurses taking up public health roles such as needs assessment. This is supported by targets within *Valuing People*, in which it is a stated objective that all people with learning disabilities need to register with a general practitioner. Learning disability nurses could be asked to monitor performance in this area, probably as part of their health facilitation remit. The Welsh Assembly Government (2002) document calls on learning disability nurses to play a role in influencing others and challenging public attitudes, though it is not specific in which capacity nurses would do this. Finally, the NHS Scotland (2002) document contains recommendations about the leadership and co-ordinating role for the learning disability nurse. It calls on NHS Boards to create more leadership and consultant nurse posts in learning disability. However, their role might be limited because the document envisages learning disability nurses being based in primary health care settings in the future. This potentially places learning disability nurses in an influential position within public health, though there is a query over the extent to which nurses could maintain links with professional colleagues and other members of learning disability teams.

In spite of the support for learning disability nurses becoming leaders and co-ordinators of services, research also highlights their reluctance to take on these roles. Nurses in Norman *et al'*.s (1996) study reported that they did not want to lose contact with service users and perceived managerial roles as being 'desk bound' occupations. This was also found by Alaszewski *et al.* (2001). This may not be unusual: most of the nurses interviewed by the researchers were in posts providing face-to-face care and support and, if they were enjoying those roles, it is unlikely that they would want to move into managerial posts. Managerial posts also convey images of bureaucracy and the need to conserve resources, which are unattractive and anathema to practising nurses. On the other hand, if learning disability nurses are serious about wanting to maintain a 'hands-on' component in their role, then they face a dilemma. In other words, improvement in services will never be brought about unless learning disability nurses grasp the challenges of leadership and co-ordination roles.

This section cannot be completed without a brief discussion of who will manage and lead learning disability nurses in the future. The many changes in services for people with learning disabilities over the past three decades, and the strengthening of multidisciplinary team work, has meant that learning disability nurses have become used to being managed and from a range of sources. It appears that in the future there will be more of the same. However, this does not mean that learning disability nurses should not strive to learn how to be better leaders and managers and learn how to exercise leadership in new ways that particularly suit learning disability nurses and their history. This includes assuming the leadership of all learning disability nurses and helping them to connect with each other in order to develop a shared vision of their future (Turnbull, 1999).

Conclusion

It has only been possible to provide a brief discussion of factors that are likely to influence the practice of learning disability nurses in the future, and whether the context of practice is likely to be supportive of learning disability nurses. Although there seem to be several pitfalls, there is an equal number of opportunities for the learning disability nurse. Of course, it is impossible to be certain of what the future will bring and, specifically, how practice needs to change. In the past three decades at least, learning disability nurses have been successful for two main reasons. First, they have managed to change and adapt. Second, they have demonstrated their relevance to the needs and aspirations of people with learning disabilities and their families. Third, although they have primarily worked in health service organisations, learning disability nurses have retained both health and social care aspects of their practice. Whether this will be sufficient to sustain practice into the future remains to be seen.

References

Alaszewski, A., Motherby, E., Gates, B., Ayer, S. & Manthorpe, J. (2001) *Diversity and Change: The Changing Roles and Education of Learning Disability Nurses.* English National Board, London.

Alderwick, G., Bratt, A., Rouff, C. & Sandford, E. (1998) Cinderella is coming home. *Learning Disability Practice*, **1**(2), 21–3.

Bending, M. (2001) One-to-one. *Learning Disability Practice*, **4**(4), 18–21.

Blackmore, R. (2001) Advocacy in nursing: perceptions of learning disability nurses. *Journal of Learning Disabilities*, **5**(3), 221–34.

Brown, J. (1994) *Analysis of the Responses to the Consensus Statement on the Future of the Specialist Nurse Practitioner in Learning Disabilities.* University of York, Department of Social Policy and Social Work, York.

Clifton, M., Shaw, I. & Brown, J. (1992) *The Transferability of Mental Handicap Nursing Skills from Hospital to Community.* University of York, Department of Social Policy and Social Work, York.

Department of Health (1997) *The NHS – Modern, Dependable.* Department of Health, London.

Department of Health (2001) *Valuing People: A New Strategy for Learning Disability in the 21st Century.* Department of Health, London.

Department of Health (2003) *Agenda for Change: A New System of Pay for the NHS.* Department of Health, London.

Hogg, J., Lucchino, R., Wang, K. & Janicki, M. (2000) *Healthy Ageing – Adults with Intellectual Disabilities: Ageing and Social Policy.* World Health Organization, Geneva.

Iles, I.K. (2003) Becoming a learning organisation: a precondition for person-centred services to people with learning difficulties. *Journal of Learning Disabilities*, **7**(1), 65–77.

James, A. (1994) *Managing to Care: Public Services and the Market.* Longman, London.

MENCAP (2003) *Out of Sight, Out of Mind.* MENCAP, London.

National Health Service Scotland (2002) *Promoting Health, Supporting Inclusion. The National Review of the Contribution of all Nurses and Midwives to the Care and Support of People with Learning Disabilities.* NHS Scotland, Edinburgh.

Norman, I., Redfern, S., Bodley, D., Holroyd, S., Smith, C. & White, E. (1996) *The Changing Educational Needs of Mental Health and Learning Disability Nurses.* English National Board, London.

Northfield, J. & Turnbull, J. (2001) Experiences from cancer services. In Hogg, J.,

Northfield, J. & Turnbull, J. (eds), *Cancer and People with Learning Disabilities*. British Institute of Learning Disabilities, Kidderminster.

Nursing Times (1991) Colleges fail to fill mental handicap courses. *Nursing Times News*, **87**(23), 7.

Nursing Times (2003) Nurses win £100 million for ongoing training. *Nursing Times Recruitment*, **5**, 6.

Parahoo, P. & Barr, O. (1994) A profile of learning disability nurses. *Nursing Standard*, **8**(42), 35–9.

Proctor, S. (2000) *Caring for Health*. MacMillan, Basingstoke.

Race, D. (1995) Historical development of service provision. In Malin, N. (ed.), *Services for People with Learning Disabilities*. Routledge, London.

Stewart, D. & Todd, M. (2001) Role and contribution of nurses for learning disabilities: a local study in a county of the Oxford–Anglia region. *British Journal of Learning Disabilities*, **29**, 145–50.

Turnbull, J. (1999) Who will lead the way? *Learning Disability Practice*, **2**(2), 12–16.

Turnbull, J. (2000) An opportunity for learning. *Learning Disability Practice*, **3**(4), 3.

Turnbull, J. (2002) Managing to change the way we manage to change. In Howkins, E. & Thronton, C. (eds), *Managing and Leading Innovation in Health Care*. Ballière Tindall, London.

Welsh Assembly Government (2002) *Inclusion, Partnership and Innovation: A Framework for Realising the Potential of Learning Disability Nursing in Wales*. Welsh Assembly Government, Cardiff.

Wolverson, M. (2000) On reflection. *Learning Disability Practice*, **3**(2), 24–7.

Index